*FAST*FUEL FOOD FOR TRIATHLON SUCCESS

FAST FUEL
FOOD FOR TRIATHLON SUCCESS

Recipes and Nutrition Plans to
Help You Achieve Your Goals

RENEE MCGREGOR

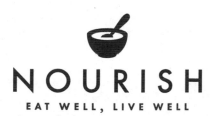

NOURISH
EAT WELL, LIVE WELL

Fast Fuel: Food for Triathlon Success
Renee McGregor

Some of the material in this book was
previously published in the UK and USA
in 2015 as *Training Food*

This edition published in the UK and USA
in 2016 by Nourish, an imprint of Watkins
Media Limited
19 Cecil Court
London WC2N 4HE

enquiries@nourishbooks.com

Publisher: Jo Lal
Managing Editor: Rebecca Woods
Editors: Dawn Bates, Judy Barratt and
  Wendy Hobson
Designer: Clare Thorpe
Production: Uzma Taj

A CIP record for this book is available from
the British Library

ISBN: 978-1-84899-303-7

10 9 8 7 6 5 4 3 2 1

Typeset in Clavo and Avant Garde Gothic
Printed in Europe

Publisher's note
While every care has been taken in compiling
the recipes for this book, Watkins Media
Limited, or any other persons who have been
involved in working on this publication,
cannot accept responsibility for any errors
or omissions, inadvertent or not, that may
be found in the recipes or text, nor for any
problems that may arise as a result of preparing
one of these recipes. If you are pregnant or
breastfeeding or have any special dietary
requirements or medical conditions, it is
advisable to consult a medical professional
before following any of the recipes contained
in this book.

Notes on the recipes
Unless otherwise stated:
Use free-range eggs
Use medium eggs, fruit and vegetables
Use fresh ingredients, including herbs
  and chillies
Use unwaxed lemons
Do not mix metric and imperial measurements
1 tsp = 5ml 1 tbsp = 15ml 1 cup = 250ml

nourishbooks.com

CONTENTS

INTRODUCTION

This book is for triathletes of all levels – elite, recreational, young or old, experienced or new to sport. It is for those of you who want to:

>>> **Achieve your performance goals**, whether that's improving your weekly trial time, bettering your personal best time in the Sprint to Olympic distance, or venturing into Ironman territory.

>>> **Stick to a training plan** while also trying to earn a living and juggle family commitments; creating meals that ensure you can fuel your evening training session, but that benefit and are enjoyed by the whole family.

>>> **Improve your knowledge of nutrition** as well as de-bunking some of the common myths. For example, you may know that you need to eat carbohydrate for energy and protein for recovery, but struggle to understand how this translates into real food options.

>>> **Increase your confidence** by knowing you are eating the right foods to fuel your body and maximize your training, without over-reaching and potentially risking injury or illness.

There is so much information about nutrition available but not all of it is backed up by science. As a registered dietitian and sports nutritionist, I have to ensure that all the advice I provide is evidence based – that is, there has been reliable research around the subject to make the claims credible and accurate. My job is to make the science accessible. Through researching all the latest studies and interpreting them into practical application, I produce recipes and nutrition plans that work for all lifestyles and budgets.

No matter whom I am working with, I see it as a collaborative journey. I first help athletes to understand the fundamentals of good nutrition and then, with practical suggestions, piece it all together to develop a nutrition plan that works for them.

This is what I am offering you here – a practical, easy-to-follow, step-by-step, scientific book about sports nutrition, including simple but mouth-watering recipes, that you can tailor to your training needs.

>>> Chapter 1 is a practical guide to what to eat, when to eat and how much to eat. We also look at how your body metabolizes food into fuel, and how it can adapt to provide fuel for different levels of training intensity.

>>> Chapter 2 shows the different fuelling requirements for different distances and training intensities and how making the right nutritional choices will benefit you. This section also includes sample menu plans, using the recipes from the book to demonstrate practically how to make appropriate choices.

>>> Chapter 3 highlights the importance of maintaining the well-oiled machine we call our body; it looks at issues relating to injury, illness and over-reaching and demonstrates how the right nutrition can combat these potential problems.

There are fun and practical quick tips throughout the book that deliver up-to-date and evidence-based sports nutrition in bitesize and accessible ways.

CHAPTER 1
FUELLING
BASICS

FROM SPRINT TO IRONMAN

There is so much hype surrounding sports nutrition these days; the science is evolving, with an increasing number of studies proving that nutrition plays an important part in performance gains. This chapter will help you to understand why correct fuelling around your triathlon training is important to achieve your goals and optimize your performance.

You will probably have some idea of the basics of good nutrition – for example, that you should eat carbohydrate for energy, protein for repair, fat to absorb important nutrients, and vitamins and minerals for a healthy immune system. In this chapter we will look at these factors in more detail and I will explain how the quality of these nutrients, and when you consume them, plays a fundamental role in sports nutrition.

So, whether your weekly training is less than 10 hours or over 20 hours, the basic principles of good nutrition are applicable to all; whether you're a novice or an Olympian, a Sprint triathlete or Ironman, you need to begin with a strong nutritional foundation. Once this has been established, you can move on to a more detailed nutritional plan, helping to make you stronger, fitter and more able to meet your performance goals.

BEFORE YOU READ ON...

When working with sports nutrition, it is normal to calculate the nutritional requirements for each macro-nutrient to ensure that training fuel demands are being met. These are converted based on your weight in kilograms, so throughout the book I will be referring to grams of nutrients per kilogram of your body weight, or as you will see it displayed: 'g/kg BW'. Therefore, a great starting point would be to calculate your weight in kilograms. Most home scales will have conversions. Using metric values ensures greater accuracy.

THE SPECIFICS OF SPORTS NUTRITION

The main difference between healthy eating and sports nutrition is the attention to detail and the fine-tuning of nutrient delivery. In healthy eating, the ultimate goal is to promote long-term good health and fend off increased risks of disease, while maintaining a balance so that food is still enjoyable. In comparison, sports nutrition, although still based on healthy eating guidelines to an extent, is performance driven. It is about getting the best out of your training over the three disciplines, whether that's an early-morning swim session followed by a lunch-time run, or a three-hour bike ride at the weekend. Tailoring your nutrition choices to your training, including the intensity, frequency and volume, will ensure that you have:

1 > Put the right amount and type of fuel into your body to meet the demands of your training session, allowing you to perform to your best ability (we will go into this in more detail when we discuss different intensity levels of training in Chapter 2)

2 > Made the correct choices after your training session, helping your body to recover, repair and adapt

The key to good sports nutrition is both preparation and organization; fundamentally, to achieve your goal you need to tailor your nutrition to the exact training session. It's not just about energy in and energy out. By just meeting energy demands, you may be able to carry out all your training but you may not see any actual improvements in your day-to-day training and overall performance.

Making good nutritional choices will ensure that the following adaptations occur from training:

>>> Increases in strength and lean muscle mass

>>> Good consistency at each training session, ensuring you can conduct
each one to the best of your ability and progress your performance

>>> Good sleep patterns, a good mood and high energy levels

TRAINING NUTRITION

So what types of food should you eat before a training session? Training
is the stimulus that sends messages to your muscles to work at a specific
level. In order for this stimulus to work effectively, you will need to feed
it appropriately. What you feed your body before training will very much
depend on what the session is and its intensity.

Like most people you probably eat carbohydrate before you exercise, to
give you energy. However, when you go for a 45-minute swim, do you ever
stop to think about how much carbohydrate you really need? Would the
choice be different if you were going out to swim 45 minutes hard or if you
were just going for a social recovery swim with some friends? The reality is
that you would need a lot less carbohydrate, in fact probably none, if you
were just going for a recovery swim, but your body would struggle to
maintain a high intensity swim for 45 minutes, without carbohydrate.

Carbohydrate is stored within our muscles and liver as glycogen (see page
14). When your body signals that it needs energy, for example during exercise,
it converts this glycogen into glucose and transports it to the working muscle
to ensure that the level of activity can be maintained. Although your body
could get energy from fat stores, the subsequent processes to convert fat to
glucose take too long and so cannot support high-intensity exercise. This
is why it is so important to fuel your body with carbohydrate prior to hard
training such as a threshold swim, turbo bike intervals or track session.

So what happens if, for example, you have a bowl of porridge/oatmeal and then head out for a slow recovery swim with friends? Your body still uses the carbohydrate provided by the porridge/oatmeal as it is still the most available source of fuel. What is so bad about that, you might ask? Well nothing really, unless you want to lose some body fat or you want to become fat adapted (see page 73).

To use fat as fuel, you need to train at a moderate to low intensity (see Chapter 2) because this level of activity is slow enough to allow your body time to provide the energy it needs from fat stores. So if you have a few pounds to shift or are trying to become a bit leaner, you can achieve your goal with this type of training session as long as you do it in a fasted state or ensure that your last meal did not contain carbohydrate.

Some of my athletes, particularly ultra-endurance athletes, such as Ironman triathletes, like to become 'fat adapted' – this means that their body becomes more efficient at using fat as fuel and so can help 'spare' glycogen stores in longer endurance events. When you think about training nutrition, ask yourself:

1 > What type of session is this going to be? High, medium or low intensity?

2 > How long is this training session going to be?

3 > What are my body composition goals?

Answering these questions will help you to choose the correct fuel and the correct portion size.

CARBOHYDRATE

Most triathletes are aware of the need to consume carbohydrate as fuel for training sessions. There does, however, seem to be a lot of mixed messages about carbohydrate fuelling when it comes to timing, type and portion size. It is important to be aware that some carbohydrates are more desirable than others!

In general terms, your carbohydrate requirement depends upon your activity level; it is the key fuel source for exercise as it is broken down into glucose and utilized by the body to provide energy to the working muscles. Carbohydrate is stored as glycogen within the liver and muscles. It is the source within the muscle that is the most readily available during exercise, releasing energy more quickly than other fuel sources. Storage within the muscle is limited, which can be an issue in longer moderate- to high-pace endurance training sessions. Inadequately fuelled muscles will lead to fatigue and poor performance, and will potentially depress your immunity, increasing your risk of illness and injury.

Regardless of what distance you are training for, it is really important to plan your carbohydrate intake around training sessions; the amount you require depends upon the frequency, duration and intensity of your training. You will need to consume more carbohydrate around high-intensity sessions and less on lower-intensity or rest days. This is summarized in the table opposite and we'll look at it in more detail in Chapter 2.

To help you meet your needs, it is important to understand the difference in the types of carbohydrate that are available. Over the years, carbohydrates have been classified in many different ways; the most common types are simple and complex, but you may also be familiar with high GI (glycaemic index) and low GI. The glycaemic index (GI) is a ranking of carbohydrate-containing foods based on the overall effect of each food on blood-glucose levels. Foods that the body absorbs slowly have a low GI rating, while foods that are more quickly absorbed have a higher rating.

Most recently, sports nutritionists have started to use the terms 'nutrient dense', 'nutrient poor' or 'high fat' types of carbohydrate. Nutrient-dense carbohydrates are those that provide carbohydrate as well as other nutrients; examples include bread, fruit and dairy and these should be included regularly in the diet. Nutrient-poor carbohydrates provide carbohydrate but no other useful nutrients; some examples include energy drinks and sugar. High-fat options provide carbohydrate but also a high percentage of fat. Try to keep these foods to a minimum; examples include chocolate and pastries.

These different types of carbohydrate are summarized in the table below:

Category	Description	Examples	Use for athletes
Nutrient-dense carbohydrate	Foods and fluids that are rich sources of carbohydrate and other nutrients, including protein, vitamins, minerals, fibre and antioxidants,	Breads, cereals and wholegrains (eg oats, pasta, rice), fruit, starchy vegetables (eg potato, butternut squash), legumes (eg lentils, beans, peas and peanuts), low-fat dairy products (eg milk, yogurt).	Everyday food that should form the basis of an athlete's diet. Helps to meet other nutrient targets, such as good fats, protein, vitamins and minerals.
Nutrient-poor carbohydrate	Foods and fluids that contain carbohydrate but minimal or no other nutrients.	All sugars (eg dextrose, sucrose, agave nectar, honey, molasses etc), soft drinks, energy drinks, lollies, carbohydrate gels, sports drinks and cordials, any type of white bread.	Shouldn't be a major part of the everyday diet but may provide a compact carbohydrate source around training.
High-fat carbohydrate	Foods that contain carbohydrate but are high in fat	Pastries, cakes, chips, crisps and chocolate.	Occasional foods that are best not consumed around training sessions.

TABLE 1.1 Types of carbohydrate

It is difficult to quantify the percentage of overall diet that should be formed of carbohydrate, which is why no matter whom I work with I use the guidelines in Table 1.2 (see overleaf). However, these are ball-park figures and will vary from individual to individual. Additionally, there is a gender difference: women, in general, utilize a much lower amount of carbohydrate than men for the same level of intensity. In addition, a woman's carbohydrate use will vary according to where she is in her menstrual cycle.

Exercise intensity	Situation	Carbohydrate targets for men	Carbohydrate targets for women
Light	Low-intensity or skill-based activities, such as plyometrics or movement patterns; core work or exercising less than three times per week	3–5g/kg BW	2–4g/kg BW
Moderate	Running for about an hour a day at a steady pace that enables you to have a conversation	5–7g/kg BW	3–5g/kg BW
High	Running at moderate–high intensity for 1–3 hours a day, including double days	6–10g/kg BW	5–7g/kg BW
Very high	Extreme running – moderate–high-intensity, or long runs (20 miles plus) back to back for several days	8–12g/kg BW	8g/kg BW

TABLE 1.2 Carbohydrate intake requirements for different training intensities

So, for a moderately active 60kg/132lb adult, who trains for 30–45-minutes across all three disciplines, three times per week, this works out to be 3 x 60g = 180g of carbohydrate a day. I recommend that you derive this carbohydrate solely from nutrient-dense foods (see Table 1.1). Even within this group, certain foods will make the carbohydrate go further: 100g/3½oz rolled oats provides 60g of carbohydrate but 100g/3½oz of butternut squash only provides 20g. You would need to eat 300g/10½oz of squash to provide 60g. Here are some other examples:

>>> 100g/3½oz wholemeal bread will provide 60g of carbohydrate

>>> 1 banana will provide 25g of carbohydrate

>>> 400g/14oz drained can of chickpeas will provide 39g of carbohydrate

So by using more of the vegetables, fruit and legumes as your carbohydrate source, your allowance will go a lot further.

In one of my favourite examples of different types of carbohydrates, I compare jelly babies to potatoes. Ten jelly babies provide 60g of carbohydrate. But a 300g/10oz (medium) potato or six large carrots provide the same. It is obvious which option will be the more filling. This example also demonstrates how easy it is to over-consume simple carbohydrates – most people could polish off a big 190g/7oz bag of jelly babies, which would provide in the region of 152g of carbohydrate, but could they consume the equivalent in potatoes or carrots in one sitting?

Having said that, in certain training situations, jelly babies may be the preferred fuel. For example, you might be training for an Ironman event and doing a long bike ride with some longer interval work, lasting over 90 minutes. By fuelling up with nutrient-dense carbohydrates, such as pasta, bagels or oats, you will have built up good glycogen stores. However, these stores tend to only last between 60 and 90 minutes, depending on the intensity at which you train. So you will find it useful to 'top up' your stores by choosing foods, such as jelly babies, from the nutrient-poor group, to provide you with instant energy. We will look at this in more detail in Chapter 2.

So remember, as athletes, it is important to consume carbohydrate to help fuel your training sessions. However, it is essential to choose the right type, at the right time in the right portion. We will look at this in more detail later on in this chapter.

PROTEIN

Proteins are often called the building blocks of the body. Protein consists of combinations of structures called amino acids. There are 20 amino acids and these combine in various sequences to make muscles, bones, tendons, skin, hair and other tissues. They serve other functions as well, including transporting nutrients and producing enzymes.

Eight of these amino acids are essential and must come from your diet. They are found as a complete source in animal-protein food such as dairy, meat, fish and eggs. They are found in an incomplete source in plant-based proteins; that is, they will be lacking in one or more of the essential amino acids. Examples include vegetables, grains, nuts and legumes. You can derive a whole source of protein from plant sources by combining plant foods in the right way. Some good combinations include baked beans on toast; rice and dhal; and wholegrain bagel with peanut butter. (See also pages 36–40 for information on vegetarian and vegan diets.)

In general terms, most moderately active adults, so those of you who walk the dog daily or take an exercise class once or twice a week, will meet your protein requirements without any problems. The suggested amount is around 0.8–1g/kg BW per day, with women needing the lower end and men the upper end of this range.

Let's take a 57kg/125lb woman: based on the calculation 0.8g/kg BW per day, her daily protein requirement will be 46g/1½oz.

EXAMPLES OF FOOD PORTIONS THAT PROVIDE 15G OF PROTEIN

>>> 2 large eggs

>>> 75g/2½ oz chicken fillet

>>> 150g/5oz Greek yogurt

Those of you who train more than four times a week and include a mix of training sessions and distances over the three disciplines will need protein primarily as a response to exercise, for repair, recovery and adaptation.

Protein has been a huge area of research for many years, with the most recent findings demonstrating how important protein is in the recovery phase in all sports and not just weight training, as previously thought. When you train, especially for endurance events such as Olympic distance, Half or Full Ironman, or during very high intensity training such as track, turbo or threshold swims, there is an increase in the breakdown of protein in the muscle. By ensuring good protein choices throughout the day, you will help to counteract this and remain in a positive protein balance (so there is more protein available than will be broken down during training).

So how much protein does a triathlete actually need? The latest guidelines recommend something I call protein pulsing, where protein is consumed more frequently throughout the day rather than as a large amount straight after exercise. This has been based on scientific findings demonstrating that our bodies can only absorb and utilize a certain amount of protein at any given time. It works on the principle that you need to consume up to 0.4g/kg BW from your three daily meals. For most triathletes this will equate to around 20-30g of protein.Those of you who also include weight training would also benefit from an additional 0.4g/kg BW portion before you go to bed to enhance your recovery.

EXAMPLES OF FOOD PORTIONS THAT PROVIDE 20G PROTEIN

>>> 3 large eggs

>>> 100g/3½oz salmon fillet

>>> 200g/7oz tofu

>>> 80g/2¾oz pork loin

>>> 1 x 400g/14oz can baked beans in tomato sauce

>>> 100g/3½oz chicken fillet

This can then be additionally supplemented with 10g protein portions as snacks through the day. Good examples include:

>>> 50g/1¾oz almonds

>>> 15g/½oz beef jerky

>>> 300ml/10½fl oz glass of milk

>>> 100g/3½oz Greek yogurt

Choosing a protein snack over a carb one is particularly useful if you are trying to watch your weight as protein helps to keep you full for longer and prevents blood sugar fluctuations. Furthermore, studies have demonstrated that a higher protein intake can be useful when you are trying to reduce your overall energy intake, as it helps to prevent the loss of lean muscle mass. The aim is to maintain as much lean muscle mass as possible as this is metabolically active and helps to continue to drive the weight loss.

FAT

Contrary to popular belief, not all fat is bad for you! In fact, it is vital that everyone eats some fat to help absorb the fat-soluble vitamins A, D, E and K and to provide essential fatty acids that the body cannot make. These nutrients have important roles to play within the body.

As with carbohydrate, there are different types of fat in the diet and some are more desirable than others!

Saturated fat is the kind of fat found in animal products; examples include butter and lard that is found in foods such as pies, cakes and biscuits/cookies, fatty cuts of meat, sausages and bacon, and cream. It also encompasses trans fat, which is often found in processed foods. These saturated fats should be kept to a minimum in our diets. The one exception to this is dairy; studies report that a component of milk fat in dairy products such as cheese and yogurt reduces the absorption of saturated fat.

Although some fat is essential in our diet, it is also important to remember that eating too much fat can lead to weight gain; 1g of fat provides 9 calories whereas 1g carbohydrate provides just 3.87 calories and 1g protein, provides 4 calories. If you over-consume calories, it can lead you to become overweight, which will also increase your risk of getting certain clinical conditions such as type 2 diabetes.

Most of us eat too much saturated fat – about 20 percent more than the recommended maximum amount.

>>> The average man should eat no more than 30g of saturated fat a day

>>> The average woman should eat no more than 20g of saturated fat a day

To put this into context, eating two pieces of buttered toast, a bacon sandwich and a bar of chocolate, can clock up around 35g of saturated fat. Ideally, you should replace these saturated fats with 'good' fats or unsaturated fats. These include:

>>> Oily fish, such as salmon, sardines and mackerel, which are an exceptionally good source of omega-3 fatty acids

>>> Nuts and seeds, including their oils and butters

>>> Sunflower, rapeseed/canola and olive oils

>>> Avocados

However, it is important to point out that these good fats are high in calories and should be eaten with that in mind.

I generally recommend you take on around 1g/kg BW fat in total a day and that the majority of this comes from good fats. So for a 60kg/132lb athlete this will be 60g. I give all my athletes a list similar to the one below and encourage them to choose servings off the list to make up their daily requirements:

>>> 25g/1oz nut butter (14g of fat)

>>> 100g/3½oz avocado (15g of fat)

>>> 20ml/²⁄3fl oz rapeseed/canola oil (18g of fat)

>>> 25g/1oz sunflower seeds (13g of fat)

>>> 1 mackerel fillet (16g of fat)

So for a 60kg/132lb athlete this would be two slices of toast with 25g/1oz peanut butter; avocado and sunflower seeds in a salad; and a portion of mackerel with their evening meal.

In certain situations this recommendation of 1g/kg BW may need to be increased. Usually, this will be linked to a training demand/adaptation or increased energy requirements. There is a big move towards fat adaptation for ultra-running events and we will discuss this in Chapter 2.

HYDRATION – LIQUID FUEL?

Staying hydrated is essential for optimal health. Add training to this equation and hydration is even more important as you will have more fluid losses to contend with in the form of sweat.

Most fundamentally, being dehydrated impairs the body's ability to regulate heat. During exercise, this means a rise in body temperature, which leads to an elevated heart rate. This, in turn, makes your exertion at a given training intensity feel much harder and your muscles fatigue more quickly, affecting your performance and putting you at risk of injury.

A symptom not often associated with dehydration is stomach discomfort. Triathletes are already at a higher risk of gastro-intestinal problems, caused by the change in body position – from being seated bent over to suddenly being upright – and the effects of the motion of running, and being dehydrated enhances this. We know that when we are training, blood is directed away from the stomach to the working muscles. If you are dehydrated, any food you have consumed before or during your run will stay in your stomach longer, leading to gastric problems.

So being dehydrated will negatively affect your performance, meaning you won't get the best out of your training. This will be heightened in warmer conditions and it doesn't take much; just 2 percent dehydration (ie a loss of 1.2l/40fl oz in a 60kg/132lb athlete), can become an issue. However, the good news is this can all be combated if you learn to hydrate appropriately around your training and also on rest days.

There are no actual guidelines for fluid intake because it depends on the type and level of exercise and also varies within individuals due to:

>>> Genetics – some people sweat more than others

>>> Body size – larger athletes tend to sweat more than smaller athletes

>>> Fitness – fitter people sweat earlier in exercise and in larger volumes

>>> Environment – sweat loss is higher in hot, humid conditions

>>> Exercise intensity – sweat loss increases as intensity increases

So how can you make sure you are getting enough fluid? The simple answer is by checking your urine colour. Ideally your urine shoud be the colour of pale straw at all times. If it seems darker, especially before a training session, then drink! Get into the habit of monitoring your thirst levels and drink throughout the day.

One quick method of assessing your sweat loss and fluid requirements is to weigh yourself before and after training sessions once every few weeks; I use this method regularly when working with elite athletes. So if you weigh 1kg/2lb lighter after a training session and you have consumed 500ml/17fl oz of fluid during the training session, your overall fluid loss is 1.5 litres/52fl oz. In order to replace this, I recommend that you consume 150 percent of what you have lost. In this case you would need to take on 2.25L. If you were 2 percent dehydrated, it takes up to 6 hours post-training to become fully hydrated again. Adding electrolytes (see opposite), particularly sodium, to your drink post-training, as well as choosing foods/drinks naturally higher in salt, such as milk or cereal, enhances rehydration. Sodium encourages the absorption of fluid into the body and also helps retain it.

How much fluid you should aim to drink during a training session depends on the training intensity and duration, and the climate. For higher intensities even over a short duration, you will need to take on fluid if losses are high; whereas at lower intensities, even up to 90 minutes in cooler conditions, you may not need any hydration. In all cases, it is worth knowing that your body can absorb around 150–300ml/5–10½fl oz every 15–20 minutes.

So now you know how much to drink, what should you drink? To some extent the choice is a personal one, but you should take some things into consideration:

>>> **When are you training?**

>>> **How long is your training session? Will you need fuel too?**

>>> **How hot is it?**

Most of the time water should be all you need to hydrate during training. However, studies show that some people, given the option of drinking only water, are less likely to drink anything at all. So although I'm not a massive fan of artificially sweetened drinks, when it comes to making sure you stay hydrated, I prefer that athletes drink what they know they will! So if this means they want lemon squash, so be it.

If you don't need to take on energy at the same time, always go for a no-added-sugar variety of drink. If you are trying to take on energy during a high-intensity or long training session, or maybe immediately before, you will benefit from something that gives you energy.

There are numerous sports drinks on the market. My advice is to choose the one you are most likely to consume. If it's hot, or you are someone who has very salty sweat losses, you will also benefit from electrolytes. If your sweat is salty, it will sting your eyes, you will be able to taste it and it will leave white residue on your clothes and body. Most branded energy drinks have both sodium (Na) and potassium (K) salts added. The normal concentration is around 10–20mmol of Na and 2–5mmol of K. These salts help to draw fluid into your body, reducing your risk of becoming dehydrated. Similarly you could add a quarter teaspoon of salt to your DIY energy drink (see tip, below).

Alternatively, you could use an electrolyte product, which come in an array of flavours and that are usually in the form of a tablet or powder that you add to water. They don't provide energy, so can be useful in situations when you are training in a hot environment but don't actually need any additional energy during your training session. I have also been known to use good old rehydration salts that you can buy from the pharmacist when you have gastroenteritis. This is essentially the same product. Always follow the dosage guidelines on the packaging. In the same way if it is a short training session, I recommend drinking water and following up with foods that are higher in salt during recovery, such as soup or casserole, or salted peanuts.

> **Tip**
>
> *If, like me, you don't like ready-made sports drinks, make your own! I tend to dilute 300ml/10½fl oz of orange juice with around the same amount of water. This will make a drink that has the same concentration of carbohydrate as an energy drink, 5–7 percent, which seems to be the optimal concentration for absorption of fluid and energy.*

SUPPLEMENTS

When you are considering the use of a supplement, it is important to weigh up its potential benefits and risks. Is there evidence that this product will actually boost your performance? Is this product safe to use and is it stopping you from making better food choices?

Ingredients in sports foods and supplements are ranked A, B, C and D, according to scientific evidence and other practical considerations that determine whether a product is safe, whether it is legal and how effective it is at improving sports performance.

Sports foods, medical supplements and performance supplements are category A. These products have evidence to support their use in certain sporting situations and are suitable for athletes who stick to the best practice protocols. That is, athletes who stick to the recommended dose.

Products that fall into category B are those that have some evidence of benefits but need further research to clarify proof of their usage. Products in category C have absolutely no evidence of any benefits and those in category D are generally on the banned list and should be avoided at all costs.

•••

DRUGS TESTING

Occasionally, elite triathletes I'm working with require supplements; whether that's a nutrient such as omega-3 fatty acids or a recovery aid such as whey protein; or an ergogenic aid that has been shown to enhance performance, such as caffeine or beetroot juice, I have to be very careful about the advice I give. In elite sport, drugs testing is a routine procedure and a positive result can lead to a ban. A positive result can occur from a contaminated source of multivitamins. When advising athletes, I make sure that any product they are considering using comes from a reputable source that provides a certificate to prove that the product has been batch tested for any contaminants.

•••

SPORTS FOODS

These specialized products provide a source of nutrients when it is impractical to consume everyday foods. They include:

>>> Sports/energy drinks

>>> Sports gels

>>> Sports confectionery, such as chews, bars and beans

>>> Liquid meal supplements

>>> Whey protein

>>> Electrolytes

MEDICAL SUPPLEMENTS

These can be used to treat clinical issues, including diagnosed nutrient deficiencies. They require individual dispensing and supervision by an appropriate sports medicine/science practitioner.

>>> Iron supplements

>>> Vitamin D

>>> Other vitamin and mineral supplements – athletes must not assume that they are safe just because they are from the pharmacist

PERFORMANCE SUPPLEMENTS

These contribute directly to optimal performance. They should only be used if advice on dosage and how to use is given by a qualified sports nutritionist/practitioner. While there may be general evidence for the appropriateness of these products, additional research may often be required to fine-tune protocols. The supplements most commonly linked with triathlon include:

>>> Beetroot/beet juice

>>> Caffeine

>>> Cherry juice

So do we actually need supplements? The main difference between branded and real-food options is the ingredients list and the way in which they are marketed. Sports products can be more convenient at times but, as you will see in the section that follows, they are not really necessary. You can generally make a real food choice that will provide you with the same benefits, but often without the unnatural additives.

Sports Drinks
For example, Lucozade Sport, Gatorade, Powerade
Example ingredients list: water, glucose syrup, citric acid, acidity regulator (sodium citrate), stabilizer (acacia gum), preservative (potassium sorbate), antioxidant (ascorbic acid), sweeteners (aspartame, acesulfame K), flavouring, vitamins (niacin, panthothenic acid, B_6, B_{12}), colour (beta-carotene). Contains a source of phenylalanine.

Real Food Alternative
300ml/10½ fl oz fruit juice diluted with 200ml/7fl oz water + ¼ tsp salt
Ingredients list: pure orange juice, water, salt.

Winning Choice Targets

>>> Both provide 30g of carbohydrate in 500ml/17fl oz and sodium to aid hydration and although the homemade drink is cheaper, you may struggle to take enough for an Ironman event.

>>> The branded product will be more expensive but is usually available at competitions due to sponsorship so it's worth knowing your tolerance of it before a race.

Energy Gels
For example, TORQ, SIS, GU
Example ingredients list: maltodextrin, water, fructose, electrolytes, matric acid, natural flavour, preservative (potassium sorbate).

Real Food Alternative
6 jelly babies
Ingredients list: sugar, glucose syrup, water belatine (bovine), concentrated fruit juices* (1%), acids (citric, acetic), natural (lemon, lime, raspberry) flavourings with other natural flavourings, natural orange flavouring, natural flavourings, concentrated vegetable extracts (black carrot, spinach, stinging nettle, turmeric), colours (vegetable carbon, paprika extract, lutein) *Equivalent to 5.5% fruit.

Winning Choice Targets

>>> Both provide instant energy in the form of 30g carbohydrate.

>>> The gel may be easier to consume during a higher-intensity run or bike session than trying to chew jelly babies.

>>> Jelly babies are cheaper, and possibly more palatable and easier to digest as you can eat little bits of a sugar at a time in just one or two jelly babies, whereas a gel provides a concentrated amount of sugar in one larger hit.

Protein Shakes

For example, The Simple Whey, For Goodness Shake, REGO

Example ingredients list: skimmed milk (94%), sugar flavouring, colour: beetroot, vitamin and mineral mixture (maltodextrin, magnesium hydroxide, vitamin C, zinc lactate, ferric pyrophosphate, vitamin E, vitamin B3, sodium selenite, biotin, manganese sulphate, vitamin B5, vitamin A, copper sulphate, vitamins B6, B9, D3, B1, B2, potassium iodide), stabilisers: carrageenan, guar gum.

Real Food Alternative

Flavoured milk, homemade milkshakes, such as Recovery Hot Chocolate (see page 197) or Mocha Shake (see page 197), and smoothies such as Tropical Smoothie (see page 196) or Summer Fruit Smoothie (see page 126).

Example ingredients list (for shop-bought flavoured milk): semi-skimmed milk, skimmed milk, sugar (4.5%), strawberry juice from concentrate (1%), natural flavouring, stabiliser: gellan Gum, colour: beta-carotene.

Winning Choice Targets

>>> The majority of protein shakes are based on milk – see above.

>>> Some studies demonstrate benefits of whey over milk, but these gains are not significant enough to warrant the use of whey, especially from a cost perspective as whey proteins are often five times more expensive than milk or flavoured milk.

>>> Protein shakes may be more convenient in certain situations.

Tip *In a competition setting, if you know a certain product is going to be available and you want to take advantage of this, train with that specific product beforehand to check that your body can tolerate it.*

Sports Bars

For example, Clif Bar, PowerBar, Promax

Example ingredients list: organic brown rice syrup, organic rolled oats, soy rice crisps (soy protein isolate, rice flour, rice starch, barley malt extract), organic roasted soybeans, organic soy flour, dried apricots (apricots, evaporated cane juice, rice flour, citric acid, ascorbic acid, organic oat fibre, inulin [chicory extract], organic milled flaxseed, organic oat bran, organic psyllium), organic cane syrup, dried apricots, organic date paste, organic sunflower oil, natural flavours, lemon juice concentrate, citric acid, sea salt, coloured with annatto.

Real Food Alternative

Options such as Chia Charge and Nookie Bars or recipes from this book such as Banana and Nut Butter Sandwiches (see page 190), Dark Chocolate and Ginger Muffins (see page 184) or Sweet Potato Brownies (see page 187); jam/yeast extract sandwiches or dried fruit and nuts.

Example ingredients list (for a real-food sports bar): oats, butter, demerara sugar, golden syrup, chia seeds (9%), sea salt flakes.

Winning Choice Targets

>>> In a situation where it is possible to eat, such as on a long, slower paced run, real food options are always better.

CAFFEINE AND PERFORMANCE

In 2010 the International Society of Sports Nutrition demonstrated a link between caffeine and athletic performance. This has continued to be reinforced by many scientific studies suggesting caffeine can benefit athletes, including triathletes, in a variety of ways. The most commonly documented evidence is in relation to enhancing performance, but how you take it is very much dependent on the distance of your event.

In addition, the specific effects of caffeine will vary depending on whether you are a responder or a non-responder. If you are an individual who can drink a cup of coffee late at night and still sleep like a baby, you are a non-responder. In other words caffeine has no effect on you or your nervous system. If the opposite is true (caffeine keeps you awake at night), then you are a responder.

So how do we make caffeine work for us? During short races up to Olympic distance triathlon, or high-intensity training sessions of up to 90 minutes, it is most useful to take caffeine 15–60 minutes before in order to get maximal effects. This is because it can take up to 60 minutes for caffeine to reach its peak concentration in the blood stream. Caffeine can be taken in the form of a gel, cup of coffee or energy drink, but it is important to get the right dose.

Best results occur with intakes of 3–5mg/kg BW of caffeine. Studies have concluded that there are no enhanced effects by taking doses above this level; in fact, it is possible that too high an intake can have detrimental effects on performance. So, the average 60kg (132lb) individual would need about 180mg of caffeine and certainly no more than 300mg; responders should work with the lower value and non-responders will probably gain some effects with the upper value. These effects can be further enhanced if taken with sugar.

In longer events, such as Half or Full Ironman, it is more useful to hold back on the caffeine until the latter stages of the race. Caffeine is known to combat fatigue by having an action on the central nervous system, lowering the perception of effort, allowing you to keep going at the same pace for longer, or being able to increase your pace as you're perceiving the effort to be less.

I usually suggest that individuals take caffeine in the last 20–45 minutes of a long training session or race to get the most benefit.

So we know it helps to take caffeine before and during training but what about after? There does seem to be sufficient evidence to suggest that caffeine does indeed have a role to play in recovery. A study published in *The Journal of Applied Physiology* demonstrated that if caffeine was provided as a recovery drink in conjunction with carbohydrate, it improved glycogen restoration by up to 66 percent after 4 hours post-exercise, compared with just carbohydrate alone. More recent studies have come to the same conclusion; practically this is particularly useful for triathletes who have fewer than 12 hours between training sessions. It promotes maximal glycogen re-synthesis, ensuring that the individual has sufficient energy available for the subsequent training session!

However what about all the bad press about caffeine intake and dehydration? Caffeine has commonly been linked to increased diuresis, potentially leading to dehydration. However, it seems that during exercise this does not occur: there doesn't seem to be an increase in fluid losses even during heat stress. At rest although caffeine does act as a mild diuretic, it seems that the fluid you consume in caffeinated drinks offsets this fluid loss. It is now widely recognized that drinking caffeinated drinks in moderation doesn't actually cause dehydration.

However, before you all go and overdose on caffeine, something to be very aware of is that there really is no benefit in taking on more than the recommended amounts. In fact, excessive caffeine intake can have negative effects on performance. Intakes above 6mg/kg BW can lead to an increased heart rate, and feelings of nervousness, nausea and anxiety. Additionally, visual processing is affected, potentially causing problems affecting fine motor skills and perception.

SPECIAL DIETARY CONSIDERATIONS

Every year there is an influx of 'wonder diets' – high-fat, low-carbohydrate, gluten-free – the promise of 'the next big' thing that will bring potential health benefits, the body beautiful or athletic prowess, but are they the real deal or just another form of faddism? Not surprisingly, people become confused by this array of different diets and I'm often asked what are the best foods to eat for optimal performance gains. Some of these diets are backed by scientific studies, while others seem to appear from thin air. That is why it is important to consult regulated practitioners for nutritional advice, such as dietitians or registered nutritionists, who have to ensure that all their advice is accurate and evidence based.

A GLUTEN-FREE DIET

In recent years there has been a real trend towards individuals wanting to follow a gluten-free diet. Gluten has become a huge subject of controversy, with many blaming it for symptoms such as bloating, fatigue and even joint pain. Many high-profile individuals, including athletes, report benefits, particularly in performance, since removing gluten from their diets.

Gluten is the protein found within wheat and related grains, including barley and rye. It is therefore found in foods such as bread, pasta and cereals, but also in sausages and beer. For most individuals, gluten does not pose a problem. The body has the ability to break it down, as with other proteins, absorb it and utilize it as necessary.

No evidence exists that there are any benefits to following a gluten-free diet unless it is medically necessary. However, ultimately, if individuals want to follow a gluten-free diet, it is their choice. They may indeed feel more energized and less bloated, but this could be due to them being more mindful of nutritional choices generally. We should all eat less white bread, fewer biscuits/cookies and cakes, less white pasta. By following a gluten-free diet these foods are automatically removed. However, do not be fooled into thinking that a gluten-free diet is healthier. There are few gluten-free products that are wholegrain and gluten-free products also tend to be higher in fat and sugar in order to make them more palatable. My advice is to remove gluten only if you have a medical reason for doing so.

COELIAC DISEASE

Coeliac disease is an autoimmune condition, meaning the body's immune system attacks and destroys healthy body tissue in error. Coeliac disease affects the small intestine, causing it to become damaged and unable to absorb vital nutrients such as calcium, iron and energy from food. The symptoms are usually weight loss, extreme fatigue (due to iron deficiency), bloating, and very frequent bowel movements. Due to an inability to absorb calcium, those who have coeliac disease may also be at an increased risk of osteoporosis, which makes your bones weak and puts you at a greater risk of fractures and breaks if you fall. Coeliac disease is usually confirmed by taking blood tests and gut biopsies. The individual will then be put on a strict gluten-free diet, which they will need to comply with for life.

THE PROMISE OF PERFORMANCE GAINS

Some claim that a gluten-free diet can improve athletic performance. There is no scientific proof to support this, unless of course you have coeliac disease. However, being more mindful of your food choices and tailoring your nutrition to your training sessions can help. Including complex carbohydrates (see page 14), with or without gluten, when you actually need them and keeping foods high in sugar to a minimum are strategies that will definitely result in improvements to your health and performance.

Fuelling your training is not about the inclusion or removal of one particular food or food type. It is about achieving the correct overall balance and tailoring your nutritional intake to your needs. Understanding the role of nutrition and how to apply this information is key to ensuring a healthy balanced diet, and optimizing your running performance.

THE VEGETARIAN AND VEGAN ATHLETE

Many athletes consider moving to a more plant-based diet. Vegetarians eat no animal flesh, but will consume eggs or dairy. Vegans don't consume any foods of animal origin.

The reasons for choosing either a vegetarian or vegan diet could be one of many:

>>> Cultural or religious beliefs

>>> Moral beliefs relating to animal welfare

>>> Environmental issues

So can a plant-based diet really be practical and sufficient for long-term athletic success? The answer is of course, yes, but more time and consideration may be needed to plan meals and recovery to ensure that you are meeting all your nutritional requirements for both macro- and micro-nutrients (see page 104).

It is often thought that vegetarian and vegan diets cannot support a heavy training load, with many individuals believing that protein requirements cannot be met. A vegetarian diet can indeed provide all essential nutrients to support intense daily training and competition needs in athletes. Although there are still several dietary challenges that need to be addressed, with the right information to hand a vegetarian/vegan diet can be an excellent choice.

By becoming familiar with vegetarian protein alternatives, you can create some nutritious and creative meals/snacks, such as the Banana and Nut Butter Sandwich (see page 190) or simply some hummus with raw vegetable sticks.

GOOD PROTEIN SOURCES

For vegetarians only:

>>> Eggs

>>> Low-fat dairy products, including milk, cheese and yogurt, particularly Greek yogurt

>>> Whey protein

For both vegans and vegetarians:

>>> Pulses eg chickpeas, kidney beans, mung beans, black-eyed peas, lentils

>>> Tofu

>>> Soya products

>>> Quorn

>>> Nuts and nut butters

>>> Seeds

When you're training very hard, it might be difficult to meet energy requirements due to the fact that a vegetarian/vegan diet can be high in fibre and bulk, filling you up more quickly and leaving less space for energy-dense foods. By using the guidelines in this book, and adapting them with suitable options, you can be sure to meet all your training food needs.

This should not be too problematic for the vegetarians among you, as many of the recovery options include low-fat milk or Greek yogurt. It can, however, be a little trickier for vegans. Although dairy alternatives have become increasingly available, many options such as almond, coconut, oat, rice or hazelnut milk are actually very low in both carbohydrate and protein.

The table below compares the nutritional content of almond, soya and skimmed cow's milk.

	Unsweetened almond milk	Unsweetened soya milk	Skimmed cow's milk
Energy/Kcals	26	44	66
Carbohydrate/g	0.2	0.2	10
Protein/g	0.8	4	7
Fat/g	2.2	2.4	0.2

TABLE 1.3 Nutritional content of milks (per 200ml/7fl oz)

One of the best ways to recover from a hard, high-intensity training, such as a turbo or hill session, is with a combination of carbohydrate and protein in a liquid form. Milk makes an ideal choice for vegetarians.

However, from Table 1.3, you will see it is very clear that both almond and soya milk are lacking vital carbohydrates, which the body needs to replenish glycogen stores. This can be addressed by adding banana and honey to soya milk, but the low levels of protein in shop-bought almond milk make this altogether a poor recovery option. To get around this problem, you can make your own almond milk, which is costly and time consuming; or you can add vegan protein substitutes such as pea or hemp.

Plant-based proteins (see page 37) need to be eaten in a larger quantities to meet protein requirements of 0.4g/kg BW at each meal; combining different plant sources at meals will ensure your meet your requirements – try adding toasted seeds and walnuts to porridge made with soya milk.

There are a few other nutrients that may be more difficult to obtain from a vegetarian or vegan diet:

>>> **Iron and zinc:** Although iron and zinc are abundant in plant sources, they are not always readily available. Beans, wholegrains, nuts and seeds have a high zinc content, but these foods are also high in phytate, which inhibits absorption of both iron and zinc. The bioavailability (that is the ease of absorption in the body) of zinc is enhanced by dietary protein, but could potentially be inhibited by supplements that also contain folic acid, iron, calcium, copper and magnesium. Zinc supplementation or a multivitamin/multi-mineral containing zinc is a wise choice for vegan athletes, but be aware of the interactions stated above. For those athletes who would prefer to consume zinc more naturally, pumpkin seeds and hemp seeds are very good sources.

>>> **Calcium:** This should not be an issue for vegetarian or vegan athletes as long as you continue to consume 3–4 servings of dairy or soya products daily. Additional non-dairy sources of calcium include:

>> Nuts, particularly almonds and cashews

>> Tofu

>> Sesame seeds and tahini

>> Chickpeas

>> Dark green leafy vegetables (will be needed in large volumes)

>>> **Vitamin B$_{12}$:** This is available only in animal sources, so vegetarians who eat eggs or dairy produce will meet their requirements. However, it is not available in a vegan diet and needs to be supplemented. It is an essential nutrient for correct functioning of the nervous system and formation of red blood cells.

>>> **Omega-3 fatty acids:** The omega-3 fatty acids EPA (eicosapentaenoic acid) and DHA (docosahexaenoic acid) are important for brain and heart function and in athletes they seem to have a role in reducing inflammation and oxidative stress. The best sources of EPA and DHA are oily fish such as salmon and mackerel, which won't form part of a vegetarian and vegan diet. However, another omega-3 fatty acid, ALA (alpha-linolenic acid) can be used by the body to make EPA and DHA. Good sources of ALA include:

>> Linseeds/flaxseeds

>> Chia seeds

>> Walnuts and walnut oil

>> Hemp seeds

That said, the amount of ALA obtained from these sources may not be sufficient to meet the levels needed to produce EPA and DHA. It may be useful for vegetarian and vegan athletes to include an algae-based omega-3 fatty acid supplement, in addition to a good intake of the above sources of dietary ALA, to ensure that sufficient levels are met for the conversion.

RECOVERY NUTRITION

As important as it is to get training nutrition right, it is equally, if not slightly more, important to get recovery nutrition spot on. To consistently produce a high level of performance, your recovery nutrition has to be optimal.

If training is the stimulus, which you have correctly fuelled, recovery food is now needed in response to this to make sure that the body can convert this stimulus to gains.

Timing your recovery is very important, but it differs according to the training intensity and the timing of your next session. Those of you who may run double days (more than one session in the day), or whose next session is in less than 12 hours, will need to recover fairly quickly after your first session.

For example, a late-night track session followed by an early morning steady swim results in a short recovery period between sessions. To help your body resynthesize glycogen stores in preparation for the next session, your recovery food should be taken within 15–30 minutes of finishing your first training session. Ideally it should also be in a liquid form, with a mixture of fast-release carbohydrate and easily digestible protein. This is why milk and milk products have become popular as recovery choices; the lactose (carbohydrate) and milk proteins are easily absorbed by the muscles to enhance recovery before your next run.

But what if you are not running for another 24 hours or more? Recovery nutrition is still important, and there is still an important window to fill, but you only need to have the recovery food within 2 hours of finishing your training, which may well fall at your next meal.

What and how much you should eat will depend on the intensity of your training session. If you have had a high-intensity session, the recommended guidelines in sports nutrition are 1–1.2g/kg BW of carbohydrate; protein intakes of 0.25–0.4g/kg BW will enhance recovery if carbohydrate intakes are sub-optimal. So a 60kg/132lb athlete who has just finished a high-intensity 60-minute turbo session should eat between 60–72g of carbohydrate and 15g of protein. This will help to replenish glycogen stores, enhance recovery and help that all-important adaptation (see page 73). The addition of the protein helps to compensate if you don't quite meet the upper end of the carbohydrate intake, but ideally after a high-intensity session the key nutrient required is carbohydrate. Carbohydrate and protein should then continue to be consumed at regular intervals throughout the day.

Following a lower-intensity session and if you are not running again for 24 hours, recovery does not need to be as immediate. Aim to recover with a combination of 1g/kg BW carbohydrate and 0.4g/kg BW protein at your next meal. Distribute carbohydrate and protein through the day, depending on your training schedule.

Let's look at this more practically: say, for example, you will be doing a 60-minute, easy-paced run and your next session, an easy-paced swim, is more than 24 hours later. The daily requirements of carbohydrate for females will be 2–4g/kg BW and for males, 3–5g/kg BW. For a 60kg/132lb female runner this will be an average intake of 180g of carbohydrate for the day, with 0.4g/kg BW protein at three meals. Best practice will mean spreading out your carbohydrate throughout the day over meals, and snacks if needed. I normally advise using nutrient-dense varieties (see page 14), such as root vegetables, legumes and pulses to prevent blood sugars from fluctuating and stopping you from succumbing to the biscuit barrel/cookie jar mid-afternoon! Don't forget, on these lighter carbohydrate days, making good choices means that your allowance will go further.

YOUR METABOLISM

How the body converts food to fuel relies upon several different energy pathways. Having a basic understanding of these pathways will help you train and eat efficiently to ensure improved sports performance. We have already discussed how sports nutrition involves an understanding of how nutrients such as carbohydrate, fat, and protein contribute to the fuel supply needed by the body to perform exercise. These nutrients get converted to energy in the form of adenosine triphosphate (ATP) via different metabolic pathways. ATP is a molecule within cells used for energy transfer and it is this energy released by the breakdown of ATP that allows muscle cells to contract.

The body cannot easily store ATP and what is stored gets used up within a few seconds, so it is necessary to continually create ATP during exercise. There are two major ways the body converts nutrients to energy:

>>> Aerobic metabolism (with oxygen)

>>> Anaerobic metabolism (without oxygen)

Most often it's a combination of aerobic and anaerobic processes that supply the fuel needed for exercise, with the intensity and duration of the exercise determining which method gets used when. Table 1.4 uses the example of running to illustrate the percentage of energy generated by each energy system for varying distances.

Activity	% contribution of ATP-PC energy system	% contribution of glycolysis	% contribution of oxidative/aerobic energy system
Track events such as 100m and 200m sprints	90	10	0
400m sprint	17	48	35
1,500m	4	20	76
Marathon	0	1	99

TABLE 1.4 Contribution from each energy system for different running distances

AEROBIC METABOLISM

Aerobic metabolism generates most of the energy needed for long duration activity; anything over 2 minutes. It uses oxygen to convert nutrients (carbohydrates, fats, and protein) to ATP. This system is a bit slower than the anaerobic systems because it relies on the circulatory system to transport oxygen to the working muscles before it creates ATP. Fat and carbohydrate are the principal fuel for energy production in skeletal muscle.

The relative proportion of fat and carbohydrate used during exercise depends strongly on exercise intensity. You actually burn both fuels throughout exercise but in general lower exercise intensities correspond with a higher oxidation of fat; as your running speed increases, your body will become more and more reliant on carbohydrate.

We know that carbohydrate can be stored as glycogen within the muscles. However, it is in limited supply and can only fuel up to 2 hours of moderate- to high-level exercise. After that, glycogen depletion occurs (stored carbohydrates are used up) and if that fuel isn't replaced, athletes may hit the wall or 'bonk'. An athlete can continue moderate- to high-intensity exercise for longer simply by replenishing carbohydrate stores during exercise. This is why it is critical to eat easily digestible carbohydrates during moderate exercise that lasts more than a few hours. If you don't take in enough carbohydrate, you will be forced to reduce your intensity and tap back into fat metabolism to fuel activity. Fat is a great source of fuel for endurance events as it can produce energy for several hours or even days in the presence of oxygen, but it is simply not adequate for high-intensity exercise.

ANAEROBIC METABOLISM

Anaerobic metabolism is your body's way of producing energy quickly, without the need for oxygen. This is useful for sprint events. There are two different pathways for this:

1 > The ATP-CP energy pathway, also known as the phosphate system, supplies about 10 seconds worth of energy and is used for short bursts of exercise such as a 100m sprint. This pathway doesn't require any oxygen to create ATP. It first uses up any ATP stored in the muscle (about 2–3 seconds worth) and then it uses creatine phosphate (CP) to resynthesize ATP until the CP runs out (another 6–8 seconds). Creatine phosphate is a molecule found in the muscles, which serves as a rapidly available and transportable reserve of energy. Once all available ATP and CP are used, the body will move on to either aerobic or glycolysis to continue to create ATP in order to fuel the exercise.

2 > Glycolysis is the predominant energy system used for all-out exercise lasting from 30 seconds to about 2 minutes, such as in events like 400/800m. During glycolysis, carbohydrate, either as glucose within the blood or glucose that has been converted from glycogen stores, is broken down through a series of chemical reactions to form pyruvate. For every molecule of glucose broken down to pyruvate through glycolysis, two molecules of usable ATP are produced. Two molecules of useable ATP provides enough fuel for an all-out sprint for up to 40 seconds. In other words, very little energy is produced through this pathway, but the energy you do get is provided very quickly.

During exercise an athlete will move through all these metabolic pathways. As exercise begins, ATP is produced via anaerobic metabolism as there is an oxygen debt/lag. With an increase in breathing and heart rate, there is more oxygen available and aerobic metabolism takes over. If exercise intensity continues to increase, carbohydrate metabolism declines; your body cannot take in and distribute oxygen quickly enough to utilize either fat or carbohydrate, and anaerobic metabolism (glycolysis) takes over. This is known as your lactate turn point.

LACTATE

'Lactate' or lactic acid is a metabolic product produced by the body. In healthy individuals, the body will maintain a lactate concentration of 0.5–1mmol/l at rest. As you exercise, lactate levels within the blood increase proportionately to exercise intensity as the body struggles to keep up with the muscles' demand for oxygen. The eventual burning and fatigue occur because these rising lactate levels cause the body to produce hydrogen ions, which increase acidity within the muscles. At the same time, the body is trying to buffer these acid levels, but the rise in activity means that the body cannot transport oxygen to the muscles quickly enough for this to occur. As a result, overall lactate and acidity levels rise and and the muscles become fatigued. As a general rule, the more trained you are, the better your ability to clear lactate, and therefore the faster the pace you will be able to sustain before you feel that familiar burning feeling in the legs.

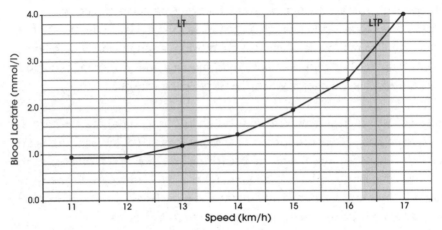

TABLE 1.5 LT and LTP indicated in relation to speed and blood lactate level

Table 1.5 shows this rise in lactate in practice for a professional athlete undertaking a test at a laboratory. At a low-intensity, easy-paced run (for this athlete, running at 11–12 km/hour) lactate levels stay low; but as his running speed increases, lactate levels rise. The first increase above the baseline lactate blood level (when lactate rises to a concentration of around 2mmol/l) is called the lactate threshold (LT). The speed that he has reached when this threshold occurs – in this case, 13 km/hour – indicates the race pace that he will be able to comfortably maintain for an extended period, eg a Half to Full Ironman. The speed at LT can be useful in defining the transition between 'easy' (below LT) and 'steady' (at LT) runs.

As intensity continues to increase, the athlete hits his lactate turnpoint (LTP). This is the speed at which there is a sudden sustained increase in blood lactate (most individuals are able to tolerate a level of only 3–4mmol/l), indicating an increase in energy provision from the anaerobic energy system.

In essence, this turnpoint signifies the maximal speed at which sustained running is possible. For this athlete, his LTP is 16.5 km/hour, therefore his race pace for shorter distances, such as an Olympic distance triathlon, will be just below this in order for him to run maximally without lactate levels being a limiting factor on his performance.

The LTP occurs at approximately 1–3 km/hour above the LT (the distance is smaller in long-distance specialists and larger in middle-distance runners). The LTP can also be used to define the transition between 'steady' (at LT) and 'threshold' (just below LTP) running. Any running performed above the LTP becomes markedly more difficult owing to the increased acidity in the muscle.

Your LT and LTP levels can be determined by completing an exercise test at a specialist physiology lab – most sports universities have these and are now offering tests to the general public. While the example used here is running, you will experience a similar rise in lactate in all three triathlon disciplines, but the speeds at which you reach your LT and LTP are likely to be different for each discipline. Knowing this information can help you to plan training, ensuring that you are training at the correct intensity for your distance. Working at specific speeds can also help to improve the speed at which your LT and LTP occur, which in turn will mean a faster performance.

RACING WEIGHT

Many triathletes talk about their racing weight – the weight at which they feel they perform optimally. There is a general understanding that the lighter you are, the quicker you will be. However, this is not entirely true and in some circumstances can prove the opposite. There is a fine line between being lighter to run faster and then taking things too far and becoming so light that you lose power and speed.

An additional consideration for triathletes is that the best physique for running may not necessarily be the best physique for swimming or cycling.

As a triathlete, you need to balance your body composition to best suit your performance. For example, if running is your strength, and you know that this is where you will make up time in a competition scenario, you may prefer to base your body composition goals on improved running performance.

The human body is made up of a variety of different components:

>>> Lean tissues, such as muscle, bone, and organs, which are metabolically active

>>> Fat or adipose tissue, which is not metabolically active

Together these components of fat mass and fat-free mass (lean tissue) make up an individual's total body weight. Being lean, ie having less body fat, at a given weight is advantageous for performance, as it improves power-to-weight ratio; the more muscle you have, the more power you can generate. So while being light can be beneficial to running performance, if you have a higher body fat percentage, you are unlikely to have as much power. For this reason, it is more useful to look at an individual's body composition rather than his or her weight alone. However, before you all rush off to try to decrease your body fat, remember that some fat mass is essential for life. We all have fat surrounding our vital organs and it also makes up 60 percent of our brain. In female runners body fat should never drop below 12 percent and in males 4 percent. Similarly, in some disciplines, such as cycling, being heavier with more muscle will be advantageous; and in other disciplines, such as swimming, having a slightly higher body fat percentage, still within normal values, may be beneficial.

WHAT IS THE IDEAL BODY COMPOSITION?

Although ideal body composition will vary according to your gender and age, the average acceptable body-fat levels for most athletes who train regularly will fall within the ranges of 15–18 percent body fat for males and

20–25 percent for females. For elite athletes, the range tends to be significantly lower. In males it will be 6–11 percent and in females 12–18 percent.

While knowing your body composition can be helpful in predicting your likelihood of sporting success, you should not use it as the only predictor. The key to being successful is to train well and fuel your training correctly. In most cases, this generally leads to a favourable body composition that will enhance your performance.

HOW DO YOU MEASURE BODY COMPOSITION?

There are many methods for measuring body composition, but I tend to use skinfold calipers. This instrument pinches the fold of skin to pull it away from the underlying muscle, so that it holds only the skin and fat tissue. Measurements (in millimetres) are taken at seven different sites, and the total measurements from all seven sites will provide a value that can be converted to a percentage of body fat.

If a trained practitioner completes this process, it has been shown to be 98 percent accurate and is the gold standard choice of most sports nutritionists and physiologists owing to its relatively low cost.

Bioelectrical impedance testing is now becoming very popular in some gyms and clinics as it is easy, quick and doesn't involve sending practitioners away to be trained in taking skinfold measurements. However, we should question the accuracy of these machines/scales as the values they produce are affected by hydration levels, food intake and skin temperature. A female client came to see me about three months ago. She had been told that her body-fat percentage was 37 after bioelectrical impedance testing. When I measured her body composition using skinfold calipers, her actual result was 29 percent.

CHAPTER 2
TRAINING –
THE ROAD
TO VICTORY

TRAINING TO PERFORM

In Chapter 1 we looked at the major nutrients your body needs to fuel itself, how your body works when you train and how this translates into a fuelling strategy. Now we're going to look at how all this fits in with your training over a given distance.

Triathlon is a sport involving three disciplines – swimming, cycling and running – as a continuous race over various distances. See Table 2.1 (below) for examples of the different types of triathlon. Between the disciplines athletes have a 'transition period', the change from one discipline to the next, which is an integral part of the race.

Type	Swim length	Cycle length	Run length
Super Sprint	400m	10K	2.5K
Sprint	750m	20K	5K
Olympic (Standard)	1500m	40K	10K
Middle (Half Ironman)	2.5K	80K	20K
Ironman	3.8K	180K	42K

TABLE 2.1 Types of triathlon

Triathlons, regardless of distance, are endurance activities. To compete successfully in a triathlon your physique and physiological make-up need to suit all three disciplines, which means you need the time to train in all three disciplines – often a challenge in itself. Appropriate training and nutritional strategies have position implications on overall performance and are fundamental to triathlon success.

Training will involve sessions working just above your LTP (high intensity) and just above your LT (moderate intensity/steady pace) in all three disciplines, as well as recovery sessions below your LT (low intensity) and endurance sessions in the individual sports. You'll also need to undertake combined training such as a BRICK session, which includes cycling followed immediately by a run; this helps the body to adapt to using different muscle groups within the same training session and simulates what happens on race day.

It is essential that you train appropriately for the triathlon distance you are working towards. For example, short intervals of around 30 seconds work the wrong energy system (see pages 42–45) if you're aiming for a Half or Full Ironman. When training for an Ironman, the majority of your training will be within your steady training zone, working between your LT and LTP speed (see pages 45–47). The more comfortable this intensity becomes, the more likely you are to succeed at completing your Ironman in your best time. Doing longer intervals of 3 to 5 minutes close to or just above your LTP speed with sufficient rest periods in between will also help you to adapt to performing at a faster speed for a longer period of time, increasing the overall speed you can sustain over a relatively long distance.

On the other hand, if you are a Sprint triathlete, your main aim will be to be fast over a relatively short distance; this means you need to train your body to work maximally for the entire duration of the event. In this case, rather than long, slow easy or steady-paced training you'll need to train in intervals. You'll do reps and sets designed in such a way that during the workout your body will increase levels of blood lactate often between 5–12 mmol by the end of the session. The main aim of these shorter intervals, as we know, is to challenge your aerobic energy system to reach its upper performance limits. You can do this using shorter reps of up to 3 minutes with 90 seconds for recovery between reps. Without sufficient time between reps for your body to completely recover, your body is challenged to work harder. You know you've made progress when you are able to repeat the same speed and time of each rep throughout the session. These are hard sessions that will accumulate high levels of lactate in your blood. As a result it's really important that you give yourself sufficient time to rest and recover between sessions (I recommend between 48 and 72 hours) and you support your recovery through your nutrition.

PLANNING YOUR TRAINING WEEK

First, let's establish your goal. Most athletes set themselves a time goal for their triathlon. It might be a 12-hour Ironman or a 75-minute Sprint triathlon, but the chances are you'll set your goal according to your time for a previous attempt. If this is your first attempt, you'll probably set your time limit according to your knowledge about what you're capable of in each event, or by comparing yourself to other triathletes of similar levels of fitness.

Your training programme needs to consider the number of sessions you'll undertake for each discipline overall. That in itself will depend upon the distance you're attempting, how many days a week you want to train, how you need to progress technically, and which of the three disciplines (if any) you already have proficiency in. Many triathletes tend to have a background in one of the disciplines, in which case if you are a runner who is keen to move into triathlon, you might benefit from spending more time cycling and swimming to build up your strength and technical ability in these areas. If you're already a proficient cyclist, you may need to spend more time building your running distance and speed and working on your swimming technique.

Always use a qualified coach or a specialist triathlon website to devise a training plan suitable for your goals and level of fitness. Expert advice will help you to avoid over-training and risking injury, and ensure you work the correct energy systems for your chosen distance.

Tip

The table below is just one example of a typical training week and is based on an Olympic distance triathlon. Although you need to fuel each training day according to the type of session you're intending to undertake, you also need to think about how all your training and nutrition plans flow together in a week. Let's look at this example of training for an Olympic distance (see Table 2.2). On the majority of days there is double training, including at least one high-intensity session. In order to progress, an

	Monday	Tuesday	Wednesday	Thursday	Friday	Saturday	Sunday
Swim	45 mins moderate-intensity intervals before work	60 mins low intensity before work	Rest	45 mins high-intensity intervals before work	1.5K swim technique	Rest	45 mins low-intensity recovery swim in the evening
Bike	Spin class at lunchtime (45 mins high intensity)	Rest	Spin class at lunchtime (45 mins high intensity)	Rest	Rest	BRICK session – Long bike ride (60 mins low to moderate intensity)	Long bike ride in morning with club 50k
Run	Rest	Track session with club pm – high-intensity intervals (60 mins)	Hilly run with club pm (60 mins moderate intensity)	45 mins low-intensity recovery run after work	Rest	Followed by 60 mins run low to moderate intensity total time 2 hours	Rest

TABLE 2.2 A weekly training schedule for a triathlon

athlete undertaking this kind of training schedule needs to keep on top of carbohydrate intake before and during recovery. Keeping carbs up will also help to reduce the risk of injury, fatigue and over-reaching (see page 113).

The following examples demonstrate what training sessions look and feel like and consider the nutritional demands they might have on your body.

TRAINING INTENSITY

There are three levels of intensity for training:

>>> Low (easy)

>>> Moderate (steady)

>>> High (threshold)

In order to achieve your performance goals, you'll need to timetable sessions that enable you to train at different intensities in any given week – regardless of the distance you're aiming to cover in your triathlon.

Planning the intensity of your exercise is important to help you determine the amounts and types of fuel you will require around a given training session. Gunnar Borg, a researcher and lecturer at Stockholm University in the 1970s, devised a scale to measure training intensity, which

 Tip

As you are likely to have fewer than 12 hours recovery between training sessions, you will need to pay specific attention to your nutritional choices during recovery to ensure that your body has sufficient energy for the following session.

Rating	Description	Exertion Level
0	Nothing at all	No activity
0.5	Very, very light	Gentle walk/swim/cycle
1	Very light	Gentle walk/swim/cycle
2	Fairly light	Brisker walk/swim/cycle
3	Moderate	Light jog/swim/cycle
4	Somewhat hard	Easy run/swim/cycle
5	Hard	Easy run/swim/cycle
6		Steady run/swim/cycle
7	Very hard	Steady run/swim/cycle
8		Threshold run/swim/cycle
9		Threshold run/swim/cycle
10	Very, very hard (maximal)	Threshold run/swim/cycle

TABLE 2.3 The Borg Scale

athletes still commonly use today. Sometimes called the Borg Scale, this rates your level of perceived effort (RPE) on a scale from 1 to 10, where 1 is no effort and 10 is maximum effort.

As soon as RPE reaches 8 and above, it becomes increasingly important that your body can access carbohydrate as its main fuel source, so that it can maintain that intensity for a given period.

Remember, carbohydrate is easily and rapidly converted to glucose to supply the working muscle with sufficient energy to maintain high-intensity exercise. If you do not consume sufficient carbohydrate, your body will have to break down fat stores to release glucose. This process occurs at a much slower rate, which means that the body can't deliver glucose fast enough to the working muscle to maintain your pace, forcing you to reduce the intensity of your exercise. (Of course, the opposite is also true – when you're training at a lower intensity, you don't need as much carbohydrate in your system.) We will look at the benefits and nutritional implications of training at each of these intensities later in this chapter.

Only you can determine how hard you are training or are proposing to train – an easy session for one person may feel like a steady or threshold session for another. Someone new to triathlon may find doing a Brick session of 45 minutes cycling, followed by a 15-minute run a high-intensity session, whereas a seasoned triathlete will find this easy.

LOW-INTENSITY TRAINING

Regardless of which of the three disciplines you are training for – swimming, cycling or running – a low-intensity session will always follow the same format: a maximum of 60 minutes at an easy pace (around 50 percent of your maximal heart rate). As a rule of thumb, this is the pace at which you are still able to have a conversation while you train. You will feel more energized after this type of session, so it's a good one to put between two harder sessions.

Some examples of low-intensity training in the three triathlon disciplines are:

>>> Maximum of 60-minute swim, any stroke – around 50 percent of your maximal heart rate

>>> Maximum of 60 minutes ride at an easy pace – around 50 percent of your maximal heart rate and building on your overall aerobic endurance

>>> Maximum of 60 minutes run at an easy pace – around 50 percent of your maximal heart rate. The run will be between 90 seconds to 2 minutes slower per mile than your race pace; it should always be slower, never quicker

LOW-INTENSITY TRAINING FOR ACTIVE RECOVERY

We know that working at a high intensity increases the acidity levels within the muscle. For some people it can take more than 24 hours for acidity levels to return to normal. Some training plans use low-intensity training as an active recovery session 12 to 24 hours after a high-intensity session. Working at a low intensity, the body can increase its uptake of oxygen, which in turn can help reduce acid levels. So, for example, if you have completed a high-intensity interval session on the turbo (stationary bike), your body may still be fatigued up to 72 hours later (how long your recovery takes will depend on the length and format the session). An easy pace for 20 to 60 minutes as your next training session, gives your body a chance to recover, while still working your aerobic system at a level that puts no additional stress on your body. This format of alternate-day training sessions also helps to reduce your risk of developing injury or illness as your body is not continually pushed to its maximum level of effort.

FUEL REQUIREMENTS

A low intensity training session has no fuel demands. Working at a low intensity, such as doing an easy run or swim, the body can oxidize a higher percentage of fat for fuel to provide energy to the working muscles; there is no urgency for the muscle to receive energy quickly to maintain a high-intensity level of work. Everybody needs and has fat stores (although some of us may have more of them than others) and they are there for a reason – to provide energy. Fat is a great fuel for endurance events, but it is not adequate for high-intensity exercise sessions, such as sprints or intervals. If you are exercising at a low intensity, as long as your body is getting sufficient oxygen to allow fat metabolism to occur, you have enough stored fat to fuel activity for hours or even days. Training at this intensity in a low-carbohydrate or carbohydrate-depleted state, such as first thing in the morning before breakfast, can improve your body's ability to use fat as fuel. Recent studies have found that athletes whose bodies are more efficient at using fat as fuel retain their internal carbohydrate (glycogen stored in the body) and exogenous carbohydrate (carbohydrate taken in during the session) stores for longer, which in turn means they can run at a slightly faster pace for longer before they hit the wall (or without hitting it at all). That said, you don't have to do easy-pace sessions first thing in the morning if that doesn't fit with your schedule. The great thing about them is that they don't need any specific fuelling strategy as preparation, and you can do them any time that fits.

So on a day when you are doing only an easy-pace, low-intensity training session and are not following up with a second moderate or hard session later in the day, your maximum carbohydrate requirement will be 3g/kg BW and your protein requirement will be 3–4 servings of up to 0.4g/kg BW a day. You'll achieve this easily if you stick to three meals a day, combining a fist-size portion of complex carbohydrate foods, such as oats, sweet potato, root vegetables or pulses, with a palm-size portion of protein, such as eggs, chicken or fish at each meal, served with unlimited undressed salad or vegetables. Snack on fruit or vegetables.

Of course, though, if you're training for a triathlon you're likely to be doing a further session later in the day. In that case, you'll need to increase your carbohydrate intake to 5–7g/kg BW, so 4–6 fist-sized servings and 3 servings of 0.4g/kg BW protein at meals, with 10g protein top up as snacks throughout the day.

Timing is important too. You'll need to consume your recovery nutrition within 30 minutes of finishing your first training session so that you start the replenishing process and ensure that you have sufficient energy for your second session of the day.

The low-intensity training sample menus (see pages 62–63) are really helpful for demonstrating how to meet the nutritional requirements for these low-intensity training days, and rest days. All the recipes, which you'll find in the book, will meet your training requirements, and they are all suitable for serving up to the rest of the family, too!

Although you're concentrating on low-intensity exercise, you still need to stay hydrated. A lot of people are unaware that dehydration is often the cause of the 'heavy leg' feeling you sometimes get during exercise. Water or no-added-sugar squash should be your preferred choice of fluids; remember this is a low-intensity session for no more than 60 minutes with little stress on the body, so the energy demand is also low – there is no need to take on extra sugar (fuel). Aim to drink 3–5ml/kg BW of non-nutritive fluid 2 hours before your session, or no more than 200ml/7fl oz every 20 minutes during the session.

EATING TOO MUCH CARBOHYDRATE

Athletes often ask me why they seem to gain weight during training, particularly athletes who are doing endurance events. With so much information on the internet and social media and in magazines, it's easy to become confused about nutrition. There is this common misconception that increased training means that you need to load up on carbs at every given opportunity. We have already learnt that carbohydrate is needed for higher-intensity/speed sessions. Those of you doing a Sprint or Olympic distance may well be doing more higher-intensity training than those doing longer distances; however, those of you who are training for a longer distance triathlon, such as Half or Full Ironman, need to do the majority of your training at moderate to easy intensity, with a couple of speed sessions thrown in. As a result, your body's demand for carbohydrate as a form of energy generally will be lower than you might anticipate.

Those of you who are new to triathlon may have fallen into the trap of thinking that as you increase the amount of triathlon training you're doing, your energy intake, including your carbohydrate intake, also needs to increase, without taking into consideration the intensity at which you are training. Over-consuming energy, regardless of whether it arrives in the form of carbohydrate, protein or fat, on a regular basis leaves your body with an excess that it needs to store. That excess becomes fat deposits. It is particularly easy to over-consume the wrong types of carbs – think back to the example of jelly babies and potatoes on page 17. Fat and protein foods have a higher satiety factor, meaning they keep you fuller for longer and so in general you're less likely to eat too much of them.

LOW-INTENSITY TRAINING MEAL PLANS

Take some time to look at the low-intensity sample menus below, which help to demonstrate how you can meet your body's nutritional requirements for a low-intensity training day; even with double sessions. They refer to recipes in the book, all of which are suitable for the whole family, while still making sure you are meeting your body's needs during training.

Sample Menu plan 1

60-minute low-intensity session

Breakfast: Scrambled Egg Pitta (see page 133) (eat within 30 minutes of completing session)

Snack: Banana

45-minute high-intensity session

Lunch: Sweet Potato and Red Lentil Soup (see page 147) with a Cheese and Chilli Scone (see page 194)

Snack: Tropical Smoothie (see page 196)

Dinner:	Easy Fish and Chips (see page 173); Frozen Vanilla Yogurt (see page 200) with mixed berries; Recovery Hot Chocolate (see page 197)

Sample Menu Plan 2

Breakfast:	Buckwheat Pancakes with Strawberries and Vanilla Yogurt (see page 134)
	45-minute high-intensity session
Post-training:	250ml/9fl oz flavoured milk
Lunch:	Avocado and Feta Toast (see page 150); Greek yogurt with honey and fruit
Snack:	Slice of Choco-Nut Banana Bread (see page 189)
	40-minute moderate-intensity session
Dinner:	Rosemary and Paprika Vegetable and Bean Hot Pot (see page 175); Berry and Toasted Almond Pot (see page 201)

Sample Menu Plan 3

	30-minute moderate-intensity session
Breakfast:	Scrambled Egg Pitta (see page 133)
Lunch:	Three-Lentil Dhal with Coriander and Chilli (see page 148)
Snack:	Dark Chocolate and Ginger Muffin (see page 184)
	30-minute moderate-intensity session
Dinner:	Sweet Potato Parcels (see page 180); Frozen Vanilla Yogurt (see page 200) with fruit salad

MODERATE-INTENSITY TRAINING

This level of training feels like 6–7/10 RPE (see page 57) or around 60–70 percent of your maximal heart rate. It is the pace at which you feel 'worked'; it is generally the performance pace you can maintain for 2–4 hours, depending on your experience as a triathlete and also the discipline of your training session – that is, whether it is run, bike or swim. Remember that moderate intensity is the pace between your lactate threshold and lactate turn point (see pages 46–47). This means that your body's oxygen uptake is at a higher level than its acid production, keeping the pH of your muscle within normal limits. If your training intensity takes you above your LTP, your acid production increases. You can't draw in oxygen fast enough to neutralise the effects of the increased acid, so the pH within your muscle falls (meaning that it is more acid). A lower pH in your muscles becomes the limiting factor in your performance.

A moderate-intensity training session will look a little different depending on which of the triathlon disciplines you are training in. Some training scenarios might include:

>>> **Run:** A moderate-intensity training session for Sprint or Olympic distance will be a 'tempo' run. This is a 10-minute warm up, immediately followed by 20–40 minutes at a faster pace, about 30 seconds slower than your race pace and close to your lactate threshold. This tempo pace will feel hard but controlled; you won't be able to talk comfortably but it should not feel as if you're racing. For Half to Full Ironman distance, steady running is vital and you will include several steady runs a week; possibly even two a day a few times a week, to help build mileage and endurance. These runs may take the format of a continuous longer run, up to 3 hours staying close to the bottom end of your steady training zone; or may incorporate, in the middle of the run, some

faster-pace miles, or even a more continuous tempo block at the higher end of the steady running zone; this pace should never feel hard.

>>> **Bike:** Moderate-intensity training rides usually take the format of a 'steady state', varying in time from 60–90 minutes in Sprint to Olympic distance and 2–4 hours for Half to Full Ironman distance; or it makes up a faster or hilly middle section within a long 6-hour bike ride, mainly in Full Ironman training. This is faster than your 'easy' pace. You should be able to carry on a conversation, but may have to occasionally take an extra breath between sentences. If you use a heart-rate monitor, it will be working at around 60–70 percent of your maximal heart rate. These sessions can be done on the road, or on a turbo trainer or spinning bike, but remember to keep to the right intensity.

>>> **Swim:** A typical session for Sprint or Olympic distance is a moderate-intensity swim session with drills. Warm up with 100m easy pace in any stroke; 30 seconds rest and then 8 sets of 4 x 25m at a moderate intensity, RPE 6–7/10 with 10 seconds rest between each 25m and 3 minutes rest between each set in a competing stroke; cool down with 100m easy swim in any stroke. In Half to Full Ironman distance, steady swimming sessions will take a similar format, but intervals may be in a pyramid. For example 1600m continuous swimming, (400m easy; 400m steady–easy; 400m steady–hard; 400m hard) followed by 60 seconds rest, 100m easy, and then repeat the sequence for 800m continuous swimming; then 400m continuous swimming; then 200m continuous swimming and finally 100m continuous swimming.

FUEL REQUIREMENTS

These sessions are harder than easy sessions, but you will still be training within your comfort zone. Your daily carbohydrate requirements will be around 5g/kg BW and your protein requirement will be 0.4g/kg BW three times a day with additional 10g protein snacks. However, fuelling a moderate-intensity session will, to a degree, depend on how well 'trained' you are. The more comfortable you become working within this zone, the higher percentage of fat you will use. To start with you will probably find it beneficial to include some carbohydrate prior to exercising, especially at the faster end of this steady training zone, and especially if you plan to train for longer than 60 minutes.

Moderate-intensity sessions don't require full glycogen stores, but having a sensible mix of carbohydrate and protein before heading out will help you to manage the session comfortably. I tend to recommend 1g/kg BW carbohydrate and up to 0.4g/kg of protein in the meal before the session. It will be more important to make sure you have some carbohydrate in store, than protein, but do aim to include some protein too.

Here are some good examples of what to include:

For morning sessions:

>>> Scrambled Egg Pitta – see page 133

>>> Breakfast Shake – see page 126

>>> Blueberry Bircher Muesli – see page 128

If you have been training regularly for a while, you may feel confident enough to do these moderate-intensity sessions early in the morning in a fasted state, but do ensure you are hydrated and keep the session to a maximum of 60 minutes.

If, however, this session is going to be 60–90 minutes or is scheduled after a hard training session, you will need to have some fuel before. Some good examples include:

>>> Banana

>>> 1–2 pieces of malt loaf

>>> 1 piece of toast

>>> Small pot of fat-free Greek yogurt with 1–2 tsp honey

If you prefer to train later in the day, whether this is around lunchtime, or early or even late evening, the key is to include a small amount of carbohydrate in the preceding meals. Again, I would recommend around 1g/kg BW carbohydrate at each meal. In simplest terms, this is about a fist-size portion, as well as your 0.4g protein portion and a good helping of vegetables or salad.

RECOVERING FROM MODERATE-INTENSITY SESSIONS

After your training session, take time to think about your recovery needs. Aim for 1g/kg BW carbohydrate and up to 0.4g/kg BW protein and also bear in mind the timing of your meal. If this is your only training session for the day, aim to eat your recovery meal or snack within 2 hours of completing your training, which may fall at your next meal, or before it

For example, you go out for a steady state run before breakfast at 6.30am and return at 7.30am. You are not planning on doing any further training today. The key is to have a good recovery breakfast, such as Blueberry Bircher Muesli (see page 128) or Scrambled Egg Pitta (see page 133) by 9.30am. It's up to you whether or not you'd like to eat your recovery breakfast the moment you walk back through the door, or after a shower!

If you are planning on a second training session within the next 12 hours and your next meal is not imminent after this run, you will need a recovery choice such as the Tropical Smoothie (see page 196) within 30 minutes followed by a meal 2 hours later.

CAN'T STOMACH FOOD?

I appreciate that some people find it very difficult to stomach any food prior to a training session; it can potentially cause gastro-intestinal upset, leaving you feeling nauseous. Some people get a stitch and others just don't like the feeling of fullness. If either of these scenarios sounds like you, I recommend that you eat 1–3 hours prior to training to avoid a stitch (exactly how long before is very individual and you will know what works best for you). (Also remember that dehydration is another common cause of stitch.)

If you already have a good endurance base and are working at the lower end of this training zone, and prefer not to eat before a training session, you can practise it in a fasted state. However, in order to benefit from the session, you'll need to be aware of the difference between this pace and your easy pace. Training in a fasted state, without any fuel in the tank, can make an otherwise easier pace seem harder – so be aware!

Those of you with a good endurance base will find that your body is actually more efficient at using fat stores for fuel and so won't find increasing the pace to this intensity as difficult as those of you who are new to the sport. Seasoned athletes tend to use heart-rate data given by devices such as a watch or app to help to ensure they are hitting the correct pace for this moderate-intensity session.

If you find eating difficult before training but also struggle to hit a moderate-intensity training pace without any carbohydrate in your system, try having a homemade energy drink (see page 25) just before you go out or even while you are out training.

MODERATE-INTENSITY TRAINING MEAL PLANS

These sample menus for moderate-intensity sessions have been tailored so that they provide sufficient carbohydrate around your training as well as recovery options that contain suitable amounts of carbohydrate and protein.

Pre-training:	Summer Fruit Smoothie (see page 126)
	60-minute moderate-intensity session
Breakfast:	Toasted Walnut and Honey Porridge (see page 129)
Lunch::	Snoked Mackerel Fishcakes (see page 142) and salad
Snack:	2 oatcakes with hummus
Dinner:	Tangy Chicken Stir-Fry (see page 160); Nectarine Compôte with Zesty Crème Fraîche (see page 202)

Breakfast:	Toasted Walnut and Honey Porridge (see page 129)
	45-minute high-intensity session
	Recover with a Mocha Shake (see page 197) and a cereal bar
Lunch:	Egg Fried Rice with Toasted Cashews (see page 144)
	60-minute moderate-intensity session
Dinner:	Turkey Pesto Kievs (see page 163) with Roasted Mediterranean Vegetables (see page 181); Frozen Vanilla Yogurt (see page 200) and Recovery Hot Chocolate (see page 197)

Pre-training:	Slice of Apple Breakfast Bread (see page 130)
	60-minute moderate-intensity session
Breakfast:	Tropical Smoothie (see page 190) with Banana and Nut Butter Sandwich (see page 190)
Lunch:	Super Beans on Toast (see page 149)
Snack:	Milk-based drink such as a latte
Dinner:	Thai-Style Baked Fish with Stir-Fried Vegetable Rice (see page 171); Berry and Toasted Almond Pot (see page 201)

Breakfast:	Blueberry Bircher Muesli (see page 128)
	60-minute moderate-intensity session
Post-training Lunch:	Miso Noodle Soup (see page 145)
Snack:	1 wholemeal pitta with Mackerel Pâté (see page 192)
	45-minute high-intensity session

Dinner: Sausage Casserole (see page 165); Recovery Hot Chocolate (see page 197)

30-minute moderate-intensity session

Breakfast: Scrambled Egg Pitta (see page 133)

Lunch: Three-Lentil Dhal with Coriander and Chilli (see page 148)

Snack: Dark Chocolate and Ginger Muffin (see page 184)

30-minute moderate-intensity session

Dinner: Sweet Potato Parcels (see page 180); Frozen Vanilla Yogurt (see page 200)

Breakfast: Breakfast Shake (see page 126)

Lunch: One-Pot Chicken Casserole (see page 158); slice of Choco-Nut Banana Bread (see page 189)

2-hour moderate-intensity session

Dinner: Margherita Frittata (see page 143); Berry Meringues (see page 203)

Breakfast: English Breakfast Muffin (see page 132)

60-minute moderate-intensity session

Recover with a glass of milk

Lunch: Avocado and Feta Toast (see page 150)

Snack: Tropical Smoothie (see page 196)

Dinner: Nepalese Chicken with Rice (see page 161); Frozen Vanilla Yogurt (see page 200)

60-minute low-intensity session

Breakfast: Toasted Walnut and Honey Porridge (see page 129)

Lunch: Avocado and Feta Toast (see page 150)

Snack: Banana and Nut Butter Sandwich (see page 190)

60-minute moderate-intensity session

Dinner: Coriander Lamb with Quinoa (see page 168); Recovery Hot Chocolate (see page 197)

ENDURANCE TRAINING

Endurance training is essential for any distance that will take you more than 90 minutes to complete. In the case of a triathlon this includes the Olympic, Half and Full Ironman distances. In fact, you should aim to do 75 percent of your overall training at low (25 percent) and moderate (50 percent) intensities. This will include at least one if not more longer training sessions, lasting over 90 minutes. Longer endurance sessions help your heart adapt at a cellular level so that you are able to maintain running for a long duration; they are more about 'time training'. Endurance training should not put any physiological stress on your body and you should be able to manage a conversation while out doing it; it is not about covering a certain distance in a given time but about the amount of time you spend on your feet, in the saddle or in the water, providing both physical and psychological preparation for your event.

Three example scenarios are:

1 > 2-hour bike ride at an easy to moderate pace followed immediately by a 1-hour easy-pace run

2 > 50K long ride over a hilly route

3 > 5–10K open-water swim at an easy pace

 Tip *During an endurance run, aim to eat a handful of jelly babies (5–6), half a yeast-extract sandwich or 3 dates every 45 minutes after the first hour.*

Endurance sessions are nutritionally demanding because they deplete your body's glycogen stores. You will need to prepare 24–48 hours prior to these sessions, taking on sufficient amounts of carbohydrate, as well as during.

FUEL REQUIREMENTS

So how do you ensure you have full glycogen stores? The human body can store around 1,500–2,000 calories of carbohydrate as glycogen. For men, this means consuming 500g of carbohydrate in the 24 hours prior to a long endurance training session, and for women 400g. Practically the most important thing is for you to take on sufficient complex carbohydrate at all your meals and snacks 24–48 hours prior to an endurance training session. The endurance meal plans given in this section fulfil this requirement, but typically carbohydrate should make up around a third of your plate at mealtimes; snacks should comprise 3–4 oatcakes or a piece of toast and a banana or a couple of slices of malt loaf. However, these guidelines will need to be adapted to your weight and body composition goals.

This 'little-and-often' approach is important as it allows for more efficient glycogen storage and causes less stomach discomfort and fewer stomach problems during a long training session. Getting into the habit of this fuelling strategy will be beneficial for race day too.

Look at the endurance training sample menus later in this chapter to become more familiar with this type of fuelling. Once you've sorted your pre-training nutrition, it is time to think about what you might need during your session.

FUELLING DURING A SESSION

Remember that a long training session is not high intensity, so it doesn't need carbohydrate as an available fuel source. If you've used the fuelling strategy I've given above, you will have full glycogen stores to provide you with fuel for about 90 minutes to 2 hours at a low–moderate intensity pace. Once your body has used up the available glycogen, it will switch to using fat stores to enable you to keep training.

When you are out training for this length of time, you will most likely face a mental challenge as well as a physical one. As carbohydrate is not a necessary fuel in these situations, I advise people to choose foods that they will want to eat en route. If you have treats and snacks that you are looking forward to, you are more likely to complete your training successfully.

Don't forget to hydrate; take electrolytes or add a quarter teaspoon of table salt to every 500ml/17fl oz of squash or water. This will help replace the salt you lose through sweat while helping you to draw more water into your body and stay hydrated. If you use energy drinks or squash with added sugar, remember that they are providing you with carbohydrate and you will need to adjust your food intake accordingly. Your body can absorb a maximum of only 90g/3oz of carbohydrate an hour, so over-consuming hourly carbohydrate can cause stomach discomfort/problems in some individuals.

FAT ADAPTATION

Time and again studies demonstrate that both carbohydrate and fat are used as fuel during exercise; the higher the intensity of exercise, the more your body will use carbohydrate as fuel in preference to fat. We have already determined that at lower intensities our fat stores are a valuable source of energy, but if we provide the body with carbohydrate prior to low-intensity activity, carbohydrate becomes the body's preferential fuel source, as it is a more readily available form of energy.

In recent years there has been a lot of interest in the concept of becoming 'fat adapted', which simply means that the body becomes trained to use fat stores for fuel even when we are working at a higher intensity. This in turn spares glycogen and carbohydrate fuel sources, so that you can go faster, working at a higher intensity, for longer during endurance events. Remember that, for most of us, full glycogen stores will fuel high-intensity

> **Tip** *During endurance sessions over 3 hours you will need 60g of carbohydrate as energy gels, jelly babies and dried fruit, and slower-release real-food options such as yeast extract sandwiches, a Banana and Nut Butter Sandwich (see page 190), a Sweet Potato Brownie (see page 187) or salted peanuts every 45 minutes.*

work for up to 90 minutes. The theory is that by becoming fat adapted, you can spare glycogen stores by using more fat stores and significantly prolong the reduction in glycogen stores.

The most recent research demonstrates the benefits of periodizing nutritional intakes, particularly in endurance events, such as Half or Full Ironman. Many ultra-distance triathletes favour a complete ketogenic diet that keeps carbohydrate intake below 50g a day, meaning that the diet is predominantly fat and protein based.

Professionally, I do not advocate the use of ketogenic diets and feel very strongly that such a regime should not be sustained for long periods of time. It is still a relatively new area of sports nutrition so there are no long-term studies to show its lasting effects on the body. However, we do know that insufficient carbohydrate intakes in athletes can lead to a depressed immune system and over-reaching syndrome (see page 113).

I tend to recommend a more periodized approach of 'training low and competing high' to the elite ultra athletes I work with. This means that they still choose to make high-carbohydrate choices around high-intensity training sessions and races to ensure that they hit the target paces necessary for their training to progress. However, for long endurance training sessions, at a low–moderate intensity, they avoid carbohydrate before and/or during training to ensure that they use fat stores only to fuel that session. Remember we know the body will use a higher proportion of fat for fuel at low–moderate intensities. If you train at low–moderate intensity in a carbohydrate-depleted state, the body will rely even more on fat as fuel. With time, training in this way means that the body gets better at using fat as fuel. The result is that even during high-intensity sessions or races, although the body will still rely on carbs as a source of energy, being more efficient at using fat will enable carbohydrate stores to last a lot longer.

Practically, this means aiming to do low- or moderate-intensity training in a fasted state or avoiding carbs for up to 6 hours before training. During the session, drink water or well-diluted squash, and possibly electrolytes if it is very warm. Aim to gather your energy from fat or protein. Salted peanuts are a good option as they contain salt, fat and protein but no carbohydrate.

Note: the observations on ketogenic diets have been done on well-trained athletes so I would not recommend trying this approach if you are new to endurance sport.

RECOVERY FROM ENDURANCE SESSIONS

Recovery from endurance sessions is extremely important. Although you may not have put a huge amount of stress on your cardiovascular system or muscles, you will have completely depleted your glycogen stores and you'll need to replenish them quickly.

A combination of carbohydrate and protein is essential as soon as is practically possible: definitely within the first hour of finishing your session and then every 2 hours after that until your next meal. Again, aim for 1–1.2g/kg BW of carbohydrate and up to 0.4g/kg BW of protein. By way of example, take a 65kg/143lb male athlete who has been out for a 3-hour bike ride followed by a 1-hour run, which finished at 2pm. His requirements will be 65–78g carbohydrate and up to 26g protein (protein becomes more important for immediate recovery when carbohydrate intake is not sufficient):

| 2.30pm | 500ml/17fl oz chocolate milk and a banana (75g carbohydrate and 18g protein) |

4.30pm	2 slices of wholegrain toast with ½ can baked beans, 150g/5oz Greek yogurt (65g carbohydrate, 25g protein)
6.30pm	3 slices of malt loaf, 50g/1¾oz unsalted nuts (60g carbohydrate, 10g protein)
8.30pm	Main meal

This type of re-fuelling is even more important if you are planning on a further training session within 24 hours.

ENDURANCE TRAINING MEAL PLANS

Below are meal plans which take into consideration your requirements for long endurance training sessions. They ensure that you have full glycogen stores prior to training in order to fuel your endurance session, and also offer good recovery choices to start rebuilding glycogen stores as soon as possible.

Breakfast:	Race Day Bagel with Nut Butter (see page 131) and Summer Fruit Smoothie (see page 126)
	Endurance activity – fuel as required
Post-training:	Mocha Shake (see page 197)
Lunch:	Salmon Muscle-Recovery Wrap (see page 141)
Snack:	Spinach and Parmesan Muffin (see page 193)
Dinner:	Sausage Casserole (see page 165); Greek-Style Potted Lemon Cheesecake (see page 204)
Evening:	Recovery Hot Chocolate (see page 197)

Breakfast:	Oaty Banana Pancakes (see page 135)
Lunch:	Spicy Steak Wraps with Tomato Salsa (see page 140); Dark Chocolate and Ginger Muffin (see page 184)
	Endurance activity – fuel as required
Post-training:	Tropical Smoothie (see page 196)
Dinner:	Tofu Pad Thai (see page 177); Coconut and Mango Rice

| | Pudding (see page 206) |
| Evening: | Recovery Hot Chocolate (see page 197) |

Breakfast:	Toasted Walnut and Honey Porridge (see page 129)
	Endurance activity – fuel as required
Post-training:	Summer Fruit Smoothie (see page 126); Roasted Aubergine, Chickpea and Hummus Wrap (see page 154)
Snack:	Latte and a slice of Carrot and Ginger Cake (see page 185)
Dinner:	Lamb and Spinach Curry (see page 169) with rice; Frozen Vanilla Yogurt (see page 200)

Breakfast:	2 slices Apple Breakfast Bread (see page 130) with honey
Lunch:	Miso Noodle Soup (see page 145); Banana and Nut Butter Sandwich (see page 190)
	Endurance activity – fuel as required
Post-training:	500ml/17fl oz flavoured milk
Dinner:	Mixed Nut Pesto and Roasted Mediterranean Vegetable Pasta (see page 181); Recovery Hot Chocolate (see page 197)

Breakfast:	Race Day Bagel with Nut Butter (see page 131)
	Endurance activity – fuel as required
Post-training:	Root Vegetable Chips with Dippy Eggs (see page 155)
Snack:	Mocha Shake (see page 197)
Dinner:	Black-Eyed Bean and Chilli Beef Burrito (see page 164) served with stir-fried vegetables; Frozen Vanilla Yogurt (see page 200)

Breakfast:	Toasted Walnut and Honey Porridge (see page 129)
Lunch:	Chicken and Quinoa Salad (see page 139)
Snack:	Slice of Carrot and Ginger Cake (see page 185)
	Endurance activity – fuel as required
Dinner:	Scrambled Egg Pitta (see page 133) and Recovery Hot Chocolate (see page 197)

Breakfast:	2 slices Apple Breakfast Bread (see page 130) with honey
	Endurance activity – fuel as required
Post-training:	Roasted Butternut, Tofu and Sprouted Shoot Salad (see page 151) with a milk-based drink
Snack:	Cheese and Chilli Scone with chutney (see page 194)
Dinner:	Salmon Pasta Bake (see page 172); Frozen Vanilla Yogurt (see page 200)

Breakfast:	Breakfast Shake (see page 126)
Lunch:	Avocado and Feta Toast (see page 150)
	Endurance activity – fuel as required
Post-training:	Milk-based drink; oatcakes with Pepper and Yogurt Dip (see page 191)
Dinner:	Zesty Mackerel Fillets (see page 170) with quinoa; Greek-Style Potted Lemon Cheesecake (see page 204)

RACE DAY NUTRITION

Long training sessions, including long runs, bike and BRICK (see page 53), are a really good time to practise race-day nutrition, helping you to fine-tune your choices for before, during and after the event. You will feel more confident on race day if you know that the meals and snacks you have chosen to eat in preparation are tried, tested and unlikely to cause you any tolerance issues. Long training sessions, particularly BRICK sessions, are an ideal opportunity to try out energy gels and drinks, and sweets that you want to use on race day. Most races will either be sponsored by a sports brand or at least have feed stations where you will be able to top up on your nutrition. You might want to find out what gels or drinks are going be available, especially in Half and Full Ironman events and practise training with these. If you find that you have no tolerance issues with these products, you won't have to worry about carrying your nutrition with you on race day. Many triathletes like to have a bento box attached to their bike in which to store fuel to supplement what's available at feed stations. Earlier in the chapter you'll have worked out what is your preferred choice for your endurance events. This may include anything from pork pies or salted peanuts to yeast extract or peanut butter sandwiches!

What you choose to eat and drink during an event is only one consideration; fuelling in the lead up to race day is equally important and will depend upon the distance you are racing.

Many triathletes know about carb-loading and for most this conjures up pictures of huge plates of pasta the night before a race. Indeed, many endurance events, in particular, sell tickets to a night-before 'pasta party'. Earlier in this section, we looked at fuelling for endurance events, which incorporated eating smaller amounts of carbohydrate more frequently during the 24 hours prior to a long run to improve your body's glycogen stores. It is always an advantage to have full glycogen stores – even for sprint races, when you will be working maximally for the duration of your race, which will quickly drain your glycogen.

For Sprint and Olympic distance, I usually recommend an increase in carbohydrate throughout the day in the 24–36 hours prior to the race. So, for example, if the race is Sunday morning at 9am, aim to have carbohydrate in all meals and snacks from Friday afternoon/evening onwards. Don't forget to hydrate too as this helps you to store carbohydrate as glycogen more efficiently. I also generally suggest having larger amounts of carbohydrate towards the beginning of this 24–36 hour period and making your evening meal on Saturday fairly light, in order to give your gastro-intestinal system plenty of time to digest, reducing the possibility of stomach problems on race day.

For Half to Full Ironman distance, I recommend a similar protocol. So, if race day is Sunday morning at 9am, I would suggest increasing your carbohydrate intake over meals and snacks on Thursday and Friday, then keep Saturday's intake to near normal levels, but remember to hydrate (I always encourage the use of electrolytes).

With either of these strategies, it's a good idea to try out meals in training. There are some great suggestions in the recipe section of this book that have had their protein content exchanged for higher carbohydrate content, in order to help fuel the muscles for the long endurance activity the next day. Some good examples are:

>>> Sweet Potato Risotto (see page 176)

>>> Punjabi-Style Aloo Sabsi (see page 178)

When it comes to the morning of the race, your breakfast choice may come down to what you can stomach: athletes I work with who get very nervous before a race often feel unable to eat at all; or long travel times can make scheduling breakfast tricky. Most importantly, don't panic! If you have fuelled appropriately prior to your event, your glycogen stores will be full and ready for action. Your breakfast is simply a top up.

For those of you who have time and no issues with race-day nerves, choose a breakfast that you have used in training so that it is tried and tested. Some good examples from this book include:

>>> Race Day Bagel (see page 131)

>>> Toasted Walnut and Honey Porridge (see page 129)

>>> Scrambled Egg Pitta (see page 133)

If you find it hard to stomach breakfast, or don't have time for it, try an energy drink and a banana or a slice of malt loaf or Courgette Tea Bread (see page 186). As before, aim to try all these possibilities out in training prior to race day.

HIGH-INTENSITY TRAINING

You'll undertake high-intensity training very close to or above your lactate turn point (LTP) and they will feel hard, with an RPE of 8 or above (see page 57). Remember, the key to these sessions is to improve your tolerance to lactate, enabling your endurance to progress and you to be able to run/swim/ bike at a faster speed for longer before the build up of acid in your muscles becomes a limiting factor. Here are three training scenarios, based on the different triathlon disciplines:

>>> **Run:** A typical session for an Olympic to Full Ironman could be: 6 x 6 minutes with 2 minutes recovery between each 6-minute effort. As each effort is 6 minutes you will be challenging your lactate threshold, breathing hard but with control so that you can keep this pace for the whole 6 minutes. If you start too hard, you will struggle to keep a constant pace over the remaining repetitions. Repeating these sessions week after week aims to help you run each 6-minute effort at a faster pace – an indication that you have increased your lactate threshold. With shorter triathlon distances, you will keep the reps much lower, maybe 10 x 2 minutes with 1-minute recoveries – this will feel hard.

>>> **Bike:** A typical session, suitable for any distance, is a flat interval 5 x 5 – this will be riding flat out so at around 80–90 percent of your maximal heart rate for 5 minutes with a 90-second recovery, repeated five times, with a 10-minute warm-up and cool-down ride at an easy pace. You could practise the session on a turbo or spin bike, or incorporate it into the middle of a longer 2–3-hour bike ride.

>>> **Swim:** For shorter triathlon distances, a typical session might be: 200m warm up at an easy pace in any stroke, then rest for 30 seconds; 4 x 25m working at 8–10 RPE with a 30-second rest between each 25m in competition stroke, followed by an easy pace for 200m; 8 x 25m working at 8–10 RPE with a 15-second recovery

between each 25m in competition stroke. Repeat this whole sequence three times. To make this session more applicable to longer distances, you would increase the length of the interval, up to 1200m at a time.

FUEL REQUIREMENTS

We already know that your body needs available carbohydrate in order to work at a faster pace. The faster you go, the quicker you will use up your carbohydrate stores. Remember the whole point of high-intensity sessions for endurance athletes is to be able to maintain an increased speed for a given distance, and you won't benefit from the sessions if you're running on low to no glycogen stores. Low glycogen will mean that you can't achieve a fast pace; or that you can achieve it to start with but then can't maintain it beyond the first 10–20 minutes when (without a stock of glycogen to draw from) your body will have to revert to fat stores to provide energy, a much slower process. This switching from glycogen to fat for fuel is also known as 'bonking' or 'hitting the wall' (see page 44). Training with insufficient fuel can also increase your risk of injury and illness (see Chapter 3).

If you 'hit the wall', you will feel the immediate shift in speed – you will no longer be able to maintain the faster pace and your body will have to slow down; almost like going down a gear in the car when you are going up a hill! If you know you are going out training on low glycogen stores, you can help to prevent hitting the wall by taking on fast-release carbohydrate – sports gels or drinks, sweets, or dried fruit are all fast-release and help to keep carbohydrate readily available.

Your daily requirements of carbohydrate will be, for women, as high as 5g/kg BW if it's an isolated session or 7g/kg BW if you're training twice that day. For men it will be 7g/kg BW if it's an isolated session and as much as 10g/kg BW if you're training twice that day.

If you are planning to do this training session in the morning, focus on consuming appropriate levels of carbohydrate in the 24 hours prior, aiming for 1–2g/kg BW per meal. Follow this up with a similar portion at breakfast at least 1–2 hours before you plan to train. If you are training this way in the evening, ensure you consume 1–2g/kg BW carbohydrate at breakfast and lunch and have a pre-training snack of 0.5–1g/Kg BW carbohydrate immediately prior to the session.

Have a look at the high-intensity sample menus (see overleaf) to see how you can ensure you meet your fuel needs depending on what time of day you are training.

RECOVERY FROM ENDURANCE SESSIONS

Recovery choices are extremely important after high-intensity sessions. Although the session is shorter than a moderate or low-intensity session, the physical exertion required to work at high intensity even for short periods can potentially deplete your glycogen stores. This type of session will also put a lot of stress on your body, which makes recovery and repair paramount, especially if you have a further training session within 12 hours. Owing to the high levels of lactate that are produced during high-intensity training, your body can take up to 72 hours to recover and it is important to take this into consideration when planning your next training session and your nutritional choices.

To prepare for a training session that is within 12 hours, consume your recovery nutrients within 30 minutes of the end of the preceding session and include 1.2g/kg BW carbohydrate and up to 0.4g/kg BW protein in a liquid form with fast-acting carbohydrate and easily digestible protein. A good option is flavoured milk or a Mocha Shake (see page 197).

To prepare for a training session that is in more than 12 hours, consume your recovery nutrients within 2 hours of the preceding session and include 1.2g/kg BW carbohydrate and 0.4g/kg BW protein as part of a meal. Try Miso Noodle Soup (see page 145).

HIGH-INTENSITY TRAINING MEAL PLANS

These sample menus will help to show how this all works practically and also demonstrate how to alter your intake depending on what time of day you will be planning on doing the session.

60-minute low-intensity session

Breakfast: Blueberry Bircher Muesli (see page 128)
Snack: Banana and Nut Butter Sandwich (see page 190)
Lunch: Chicken and Quinoa Salad (see page 139)
Pre-training: Sweet Potato Brownie (see page 187)
45–60-minute high-intensity session
Post-training: 250ml/9fl oz flavoured milk
Dinner: Nepalese Chicken with Rice (see page 161); Berry and Toasted Almond Pot (see page 201)
Evening: Recovery Hot Chocolate (see page 197)

Breakfast: Toasted Walnut and Honey Porridge (see page 129)
45–60-minute high-intensity session
Post-training: Tropical Smoothie (see page 196)
Lunch: Salmon Muscle-Recovery Wrap (see page 141); piece of fruit
Snack: Slice of Courgette Tea Bread (see page 186) and a latte
60-minute moderate-intensity session
Dinner: Bulgar Wheat Curry (see page 179); Greek-Style Potted Lemon Cheesecake (see page 204)

 Tip *When juggling your training around work, always ensure that you are organized and pre-pack portable options that you can keep in your kit bag.*

60-minute low-intensity session

Breakfast: Scrambled Egg Pitta (see page 133)

Pre-training: Banana

45-minute high-intensity session

Lunch: Sweet Potato and Red Lentil Soup (see page 147); slice of Courgette Tea Bread (see page 186)

Snack: Mango and Banana Smoothie (see page 127)

Dinner: Tofu Pad Thai (see page 177); Greek yogurt and fruit; Recovery Hot Chocolate (see page 197)

60-minute low-intensity session

Breakfast: Oaty Banana Pancake (see page 135)

Lunch: Roasted Aubergine, Chickpea and Hummus Wrap (see page 154)

Snack: Slice of Courgette Tea Bread (see page 186)

60-minute high-intensity session

Post-training: 250ml/9fl oz flavoured milk and banana

Dinner: Easy Fish and Chips (see page 173); Coconut and Mango Rice Pudding (see page 206)

Evening: Recovery Hot Chocolate (see page 197)

Breakfast: Summer Fruit Smoothie (see page 126)

60-minute high-intensity session

Post-training: 500ml/17fl oz flavoured milk

Lunch: Root Vegetable Chips with Dippy Eggs (see page 155)

Snack: Banana and Nut Butter Sandwich (see page 190)

60-minute low-intensity session

Dinner: Roasted Butternut, Tofu and Sprouted Shoot Salad (see page 151); Frozen Vanilla Yogurt (see page 200)

Breakfast:	2 slices Apple Breakfast Bread (see page 130) with Nut Butter (see page 131)
	60 minute high-intensity session
Post-training:	Summer Fruit Smoothie (see page 126)
Lunch:	Thai Green Chicken Curry (see page 138)
Snack:	2 oatcakes with Pepper and Yogurt Dip (see page 191)
	60-minute low-intensity session
Dinner:	Salmon Pasta Bake (see page 172); Recovery Hot Chocolate (see page 197)

Breakfast:	Blueberry Bircher Muesli (see page 128)
	60-minute high-intensity session
Post-training:	250ml/9fl oz chocolate milk; Banana and Nut Butter Sandwich (see page 190)
Lunch:	Super Beans on Toast (see page 149)
Snack:	Sweet Potato Brownie (see page 187)
	60-minute high-intensity session
Post-training:	Mocha Shake (see page 197)
Dinner:	Sweet Potato Risotto (see page 176); Greek yogurt with fruit

Breakfast:	Scrambled Egg Pitta (see page 133)
Lunch:	Chicken and Quinoa Salad (see page 139)
Snack:	Choco-Nut Banana Bread (see page 189)
	60-minute high-intensity session
Dinner:	Lamb and Spinach Curry (see page 169); Coconut and Mango Rice Pudding (see page 206)

STRENGTH AND CONDITIONING

So far we have talked about training from a purely speed and endurance perspective. There is another type of training that is now being included regularly in most athletes' programmes – strength training. Many studies demonstrate that strength training can lead to significant performance gains. Making the right food choices – those that will enhance the effectiveness of your strength training – will give you better results in the gym.

We know that practising any of the disciplines within triathlon tends to make you better at that discipline – and so triathlon in general – overall. However, this is effective only up to a point, with most gains occurring when you are relatively new to triathlon or the individual discipline. As your training progresses, you will reach a point where you are unable to see any further physiological improvements; it will get harder to improve on your personal best time. At this point you may choose to change distance, providing you with a new challenge. Alternatively you can focus on training your neuro-muscular system (muscle control via the nervous system), in effect improving your performance – and reducing your risk of injury – through strength training.

The next time you are out run training, look at the people around you and try to notice differences between the left and right sides of their bodies, as well as the angle of their knees and feet as they make contact with the ground, and the posture of their upper bodies as they become fatigued. The skeleton is very well designed to distribute load safely, but modern life has caused many of us to develop bad postural habits. The limitations of the bony frame mean that poor alignment leads to postural imbalance that causes stress or strain somewhere within our body while out running. Failure to address and correct the strain often means that an overuse injury is inevitable (see Chapter 3)

The term 'strength' in a training context is not limited to strength in weight training – that is the strength needed to lift weights. Rather, we can use it to describe the amount of force our muscles can produce or resist, when we lift, pull or push. When we run, we push into the floor in an 'up and down' fashion and also back against the floor in a 'backward and forward' fashion in order to move forward without falling over – so to run faster we need to push harder or more often. Similarly to improve your cycling, you need to improve the amount of force you can produce through the pedals in order to increase speed.

There are many adaptations that can occur with strength training to increase the amount of force your muscles can produce, or to produce it quicker and more effectively. These include:

>>> **Hypertrophy** – this is an increase in the size of the cross-sectional area of the muscle fibres. A bigger muscle can produce more force, or a bigger push. Imagine the leg muscles as springs; every time you contact the floor, the spring will compress and then return to its full length, propelling you forward – a bigger spring will have a better result than a smaller spring.

>>> **Explosive strength training** – to increase the speed of the nervous system signal (ie to jump faster), we may use explosive strength. This type of training involves improving the speed or frequency of the signals from the brain to the muscle, and preparing other tissues, such as tendons, to cope with high-speed movements.

>>> **Plyometrics** – one method to improve the 'stiffness' of the tendons to transfer the force produced by the muscle is plyometrics. From a training perspective this includes hopping, and bound and rebound jumping.

Strength training can be very beneficial to your performance, but you need to choose the right range of movements and the right exercises to produce the desired effect on your distance. You also need to perform all movements correctly, in order to avoid injury. For this reason, I recommend working with a qualified strength and conditioning coach.

EXAMPLE MENU FOR AN OLYMPIC DISTANCE TRAINING WEEK

It is difficult to provide a specific nutrition plan for each distance, as this needs to be so individualized. When I work with athletes, their nutrition plans are dependent on:

>>> The time available to train

>>> The level of athlete – from newbie to experienced

>>> The performance outcome – weight loss, a personal best time or just making it around the course!

>>> Occupation – some jobs can be quite physical and this needs to be taken into consideration

However, I thought it would be useful for you to see how you can amalgamate the sample menus, based on your own personal training week, and put together a typical menu.

The following example is based on a 60kg (132lb) male athlete training for around 12 hours a week with some additional gym training, so the plan also supports strength work.

MONDAY: RUN AM, CYCLING PM, YOGA

Breakfast: Before training, select something from the following list:
(Or if this is really difficult, then have something small such as 2 slices malt loaf on waking [40g carbs])

>> 50g/1¾oz porridge oats made with water, banana and 1–2 tsp honey
>> Breakfast Shake (see page 126)
>> Blueberry Bircher Muesli (see page 128)
>> 2 slices toast with peanut butter and banana

45-minute easy run

Post-training: Recover with fruit and yogurt smoothie

90-minute bike ride with 8 x 2 mins time trial efforts
(Consider taking some additional carbs on bike to have prior to starting efforts – energy gels/shots, energy drink or handful jelly babies are all good)

Lunch: Post-training lunch – recover with: 60g carbs/20g protein/ unlimited veg. For example:

>> Salmon Muscle-Recovery Wrap (see page 141) followed by a piece of fruit
>> Or Super Beans on Toast (see page 149)

Snack: 10g protein-based snack mid-afternoon, if required, such as matchbox-size portion of cheese or 50g/1¾oz almonds or 150g/5oz edamame beans

Evening meal: 60g carbs/20g protein/essential fats/unlimited veg, such as:

>> Easy Fish & Chips (see page 173)
>> Coriander Lamb with Quinoa (see page 168)

Stretching and yoga session

Late evening: Dairy choice

TUESDAY: SWIM AM, TRACK SESSION PM

Breakfast: Before training, select something from the following list: (If this is really difficult then have something small like 2 slices malt loaf on waking [40g carbs] and take an energy drink to the pool to use during session [30g carbs])

>> 50g/1¾oz porridge oats made with water, banana and 1–2 tsp honey
>> Breakfast Shake (see page 126)
>> Blueberry Bircher Muesli (see page 128)
>> 2 slices toast with peanut butter and banana

90-minute swim

Post-training: Recover with 300ml/10½fl oz glass of milk or 150g/5oz Greek yogurt with 50g/1¾oz berries and 1 tsp honey

Lunch: 60g carbs/20g protein/essential fats/unlimited veg, such as:

>> Super Beans on Toast (see page 149)

Mid-afternoon: Prior to track session: 10g protein/30g carb snack as needed, such as Summer Fruit Smoothie (see page 126) or oatcakes with Mackerel Pâté (see page 192) or crumpets with fruit and Greek yogurt
5pm: track session

Post-training: Recover from track session immediately with 300ml/10½fl oz flavoured milk

Evening meal: 20g protein/unlimited veg – some ideas include:

>> 100g/3½oz salmon steaks with stir-fry – try adding soya sauce, lime juice, chilli and coriander/cilantro. You could 'ribbon' the courgettes/zucchini and carrots and steam them so that the stir-fry sits on top and they are equivalent to noodles.

>> 100g/3½oz chicken breasts tossed into a salad – add toasted seeds and avocado for added protein and essential fatty acids.

>> 3 x large egg frittata with 30g/1oz feta cheese and vegetables of your choice; serve with salad.

>> Cook 150g/5oz lean mince into a Bolognese-style sauce, serve on top of courgette/zucchini 'spaghetti'.

>> Use 150g/5oz lean mince and top with mashed cauliflower, carrot and 30g/1oz cheddar for a carb-free cottage pie.

Late evening: Greek yogurt and fruit, followed by hot chocolate made with milk

WEDNESDAY: CYCLING AM

Breakfast: To start the day, select something from the following list: (If this is really difficult, then have something small like 2 slices malt loaf on waking [40g carbs] and take an energy drink to use during session [30g carbs])

>> Breakfast Shake (see page 126)
>> Porridge, such as Toasted Walnut and Honey Porridge (see page 129)
>> Blueberry Bircher Muesli (see page 128)
>> Scrambled Egg Pitta (see page 133)

11am: 2-hour bike ride with efforts
On bike consider taking on energy – aim for 30g carbs/hour
Post-training: Recover immediately with 300ml/10½fl oz chocolate milk followed by lunch
Lunch: 60g carbs/20g protein/unlimited veg, such as:

>> Egg Fried Rice with Toasted Cashews (see page 144)
>> Large bowl of Sweet Potato & Red Lentil Soup (see page 147)

Mid-afternoon: 10g protein snack
Evening meal: 60g carbs/20g protein/essential fats/unlimited veg, such as:

>> Lamb & Spinach Curry with rice (see page 169)
>> Sweet Potato Parcels (see page 180)

Late evening: Greek yogurt with fruit followed by Recovery Hot Chocolate (see page 197).

THURSDAY: RUN AM, SWIM PM

90-minute easy run
Aim to run in fasted state but ensure you are hydrated.
Breakfast: 60g carbs/20g protein, such as any porridge.
Mid-morning: Banana with peanut butter
Lunch: 60g carbs/20g protein/essential fats/unlimited veg
90-minute easy swim

Post-training: Recover with 300ml/10½fl oz milk
Evening meal: 60g carbs/20g protein/essential fats/unlimited veg
Late evening: Dairy choice

FRIDAY: REST DAY

Do not cut carbs too much so you have full reserves for longer training over the weekend.

Breakfast: Lower carb options, such as:

>> 3 eggs made into a frittata with vegetables and 30g/1oz feta cheese
>> 50g/1¾oz porridge oats made with water, 25g/¾oz whey protein and 50g/1¾oz frozen berries
>> Scrambled Egg Pitta (see page 133)
>> Buckwheat pancakes (see page 134 but use Greek yogurt for an extra protein hit)

Mid-morning: 10g protein choice snack
Lunch: 60g carbs/20g protein/essential fats/unlimited salad or veg
Mid-afternoon: 10g protein/35g carbs
Evening meal: 60g carbs/20g protein/unlimited veg
Late evening: Recovery Hot Chocolate (see page 197) and apple slices with peanut butter

SATURDAY: SWIM & RUN AM

Breakfast: Start the day with one of the following:
(Or if this is really difficult, then have something small like 2 slices malt loaf on waking [40g carbs] and take an energy drink to use during session [30g carbs])

>> Toasted Walnut and Honey Porridge (see page 129)
>> Breakfast Shake (see page 126)
>> Blueberry Bircher Muesli (see page 128)

90-minute swim followed by 45-minute hard run
Immediately post-swim prior to run: energy gels or shots/
cubes or 500ml/17fl oz energy drink – you will need this to
ensure you can hit paces
Post-training: Recover with 500ml/17fl oz chocolate milk
Lunch: 60g carbs/20g protein/unlimited veg, such as:

>> Miso Noodle Soup (see page 145)

Mid-afternoon: 10g protein based snack if needed
Evening meal: 20g protein/unlimited veg
Late evening: Greek yogurt with fruit and hot chocolate made with milk.

SUNDAY: SWIM AM, TURBO SESSION PM

45–60 minute easy swim
Breakfast: This swim session can be done in a fasted state but recover
with 70g carbs/20g protein for breakfast
Lunch: 60g carbs/20g protein/essential fats/unlimited salad or veg
Pre-training: Prior to bike top up with 35g carbs
2.5–3-hour turbo session
During turbo session, aim for 30g carbs per hour
Post-training: Recover with 60g carbs/20g protein
Evening meal: 60g carbs/20g protein/unlimited veg
Late evening: Greek yogurt with fruit and hot chocolate made with milk

CHAPTER 3
FINE-TUNING YOUR BODY

TROUBLESHOOTING COMPLAINTS

The human body is extremely efficient and clever, but it's not perfect. Although participating in sport is important for good health, sport itself is not always beneficial for our bodies. Indeed, rates of injury are usually high in athletes. Whether it is a twisted joint, a pulled muscle/ligament or something more serious, training puts a huge strain on the body and, inevitably, can lead to overuse and injury.

Nutrition is a continually evolving science, with new studies and research being published on a daily basis. An area that is of real interest to researchers is how nutrition can impact on injury prevention and how it can improve recovery rates from injury. As with all studies, there are mixed results and, although further research is required, overall there do seem to be some key nutritional strategies that may be beneficial.

In this chapter we will look at some common issues associated with triathlon, the stresses they can potentially cause your body and how nutrition can help to restore balance.

COMMON COMPLAINTS

Training is a time-consuming business. Whether you are an elite athlete who needs to commit to double days of training or a recreational athlete who is trying to fit a lunchtime run around work and family commitments, it is inevitable that sometimes you might take shortcuts. Some examples are:

>>> Not warming up or cooling down sufficiently before training, which can lead to poor technique. For example, by not engaging your glutes, a key muscle in

triathlon performance, you will be more dependent on your hamstrings
and this may ultimately cause an overuse injury

>>> Being disorganized and so having poor nutritional options available
either side of your training

These shortcuts may leave your body feeling unbalanced and vulnerable.
You may also choose to ignore early symptoms, which can potentially
become something more serious further down the line. These symptoms
might include:

>>> Pain

>>> Fatigue

>>> Poor sleep patterns

>>> Dizziness

>>> Shortness of breath

>>> Skipping menstruation

>>> A change in heart rate at rest, but also during running

In all these cases, addressing the issue early can help to prevent longer-term
problems and, in most cases, the problem is usually quite easy to fix!

INJURY PREVENTION

There are many things you can do to help prevent injury and many triathletes are familiar with the four Rs:

1 > Rehydrate – sweating causes a loss of water and electrolytes, so make sure you drink water before, during and after exercise to avoid dehydration.

2 > Replenish – stored carbohydrate (glycogen) is the primary fuel for muscles during exercise. It is important to consume carbohydrate after exercise to replace depleted stores, but be guided by the intensity of your training session (see Chapter 2).

3 > Repair – muscle is broken down during exercise so you need to eat high-quality protein after exercise to rebuild muscle tissue.

4 > Reinforce – during exercise your immune system becomes compromised as a result of cell damage and inflammation. To keep a strong immune system, you should refuel with nutritious, fresh foods.

You can see, then, that nutrition plays a huge part in injury prevention. It is also useful to help your body to stay in alignment by strengthening potential weak areas within it.

Tip *I also think there is a fifth R – Rest. We will look at this in the context of overtraining later in this chapter.*

NUTRITION FOR SORE, TIRED OR INJURED BODIES

One way to help avoid injury is to organize your nutrition either side of your training so that you are meeting your requirements. Hopefully by now, having read through this book so far, you will have a good understanding of how to do that, but there are some further nutritional strategies you may find useful. An area of huge interest and research is how specific nutrients, such as those in beetroot or tart cherries (see page 102), have a role to play in recovery, helping to return the body to an optimal state prior to the next training session.

SORE MUSCLES

A common phenomenon in athletes is DOMS, or delayed onset muscle soreness, especially in those who have taken on a new form of training, such as adding strength to weekly training in the three disciplines, or those who have trained or competed particularly hard. The soreness is most commonly felt 24–72 hours after the exercise. This is the result of micro-trauma, which is mechanical damage at a very small scale to the exercised muscles, leading to inflammation and oxidative stress. Oxidative stress is the term used to describe free-radical damage to proteins, membranes and genes. Studies have shown that although exercise is good for us, it does also increase the levels of free radicals in our body.

Usually if you repeat a certain exercise pattern sufficiently, your body will get used to it and the soreness will stop. However, we also know that to improve performance, muscles need to be 'overloaded' continually and so DOMS is a training inevitability from time to time.

There has been a lot of research into ways in which we can reduce inflammation and oxidative stress on the body, with the best findings coming from the use of powerful antioxidants. Some examples include:

>>> Curcumin – found in cumin

>>> Isoflavanoids – found in soya beans

>>> Vitamin C

With the most evidence stacking up in the use of:

>>> Polyphenols – most of the data has come from studies using tart cherry juice, which did seem to show a significant reduction in inflammatory markers in endurance athletes after strenuous sessions; I recommend tart cherry juice/ capsules or shots after all high-intensity training or races as a way to reduce oxidative stress on the body. You can buy these at health food stores or online.

As is always the case when it comes to research, we need further studies to help us decide on dosages and timings for optimal benefits. Triathletes can also benefit from increasing their intake of food-derived antioxidants – quite simply, you can eat more fruit, vegetables, herbs and spices (see the Nepalese Chicken recipe on page 161 for one of many spicy recipes).

AN INJURED BODY

The most important thing to remember when you are injured is that you need to rest. Depending on the severity of your injury, you may need as little as a few days to over 6 months. Being injured is very frustrating, especially when training has been going well. However, it is also a good time to reflect and work out how you can reduce your risk of the same injury occuring again:

>>> Did you ignore signs of pain and so keep going when you should have rested?

>>> Did you fuel and recover appropriately after each training session?

>>> Did you take sufficient rest between your training sessions?

Nutrition can also be instrumental in your recovery and return to exercise. A lot of athletes understandably worry about weight gain when they become injured. Research has demonstrated that decreasing your overall energy intake, but increasing your protein intake (to as high as 2.3g/kg BW daily) is a useful way to recover without gaining weight.

Protein has a high satiety factor, so it helps you to feel full while limiting your overall energy intake. Additionally, protein has demonstrated a role in repair of the damaged area. With bone injuries, such as a stress fracture, supplementing with vitamin D (see page 107) has been shown to be effective; and new research emerging is also looking at the role of vitamin C and collagen as supplements.

A TIRED BODY

When you are training hard, you are bound to feel some residual fatigue. However, if tiredness does not disappear after a few days' rest, it is important to take note and consider what else could be contributing. Ask yourself:

>>> Have I increased or changed my training significantly recently?

>>> Am I taking enough rest or active recovery time between hard or long sessions?

>>> Am I recovering appropriately nutritionally?

>>> Am I hydrated?

>>> Am I eating enough before I train?

>>> Is it possible I am coming down with a virus or other illness?

If your answers to these questions don't seem to reveal what might be contributing to your fatigue, consider whether there are other medical or nutritional reasons that could be at the root. We have already seen that a vitamin-D deficiency is linked to chronic fatigue and poor muscle recovery. Similarly deficiencies in other micro-nutrients can pose problems.

ESSENTIAL MICRONUTRIENTS

Don't imagine that the prefix 'micro' means these nutrients have only small effects and are therefore less significant for your wellbeing than macronutrients. Micro means that we need to consume them in 'micro' amounts, but they are no less essential to good health. Examples are:

>>> Vitamins – A, B, C, D, E and K

>>> Minerals – calcium, iron and phosphorus

>>> Electrolytes – sodium and potassium

>>> Trace elements – iodine, zinc and magnesium

Micronutrients are essential for many metabolic processes within the body, and although we can manufacture a few of them within the body, most have to come from the diet. Most function as co-enzymes or co-factors within the body – that is, they aid enzymes and proteins in their function. For example, the B-vitamins are very important for carbohydrate and fat metabolism, while vitamin C, along with zinc, is important for a healthy immune system;

you need magnesium and calcium for good muscle contraction. Each and every micronutrient has a significant part to play in your training success.

This begs the question, do you need to supplement your intake to make sure you meet your requirements? The bottom line is that if you eat a well-balanced diet that includes whole grains, vegetables, meat, fish and dairy you will have no problem in getting everything you need.

And, do athletes have higher requirements of micronutrients? The jury is out on this one. Some studies show that there are enhanced requirements in athletes as a result of an increase in free-radical damage in frequently trained muscles. However, no study has shown an absolute link between improved sporting performance and a diet high in antioxidants. Overall, though, if you are a very physically active person (such as an athlete), you will naturally be taking in more food, because you need the fuel. As long as this fuel is well-balanced and nutrient-rich and not made up of empty calories, you will naturally meet your increased antioxidant requirements without needing to resort to supplements.

That said, in some individuals, exercise, particularly at increased volumes and intensities, leads to elevated requirements of iron (see below) and a deficiency in important micronutrients such as vitamin D. This is linked to chronic fatigue and poor muscle recovery.

IRON

Your body needs iron to make haemoglobin, which is the protein that transfers oxygen around the body. If iron levels become low, either because your diet is providing too little or because you are losing iron excessively, you may develop iron-deficiency anaemia.

An inadequate intake of iron is possible if you are following a restricted diet for weight loss, or because you are a vegan or vegetarian (see page 36); excessive losses can happen during menstruation in female athletes, but have also been linked to an increased breakdown in red blood cells in some athletes, particularly those where running is involved.

Why is iron deficiency such a big deal? It becomes an issue because if there is not enough iron in the body, the body struggles to make haemoglobin, which in turn means that lower levels of oxygen can be transported around the body. This will not only make you feel pretty lousy, but also have an impact on your overall performance. Common symptoms of iron deficiency include:

>>> Feeling tired all the time

>>> Being short of breath, even just going up the stairs

>>> Poor performance in training

>>> Dizziness

>>> Looking pale

>>> Loss of appetite

>>> Bluish tinted dark circles around the eyes

>>> Increased prevalence of infections

If you have any of these symptoms, talk them through with your GP, who can do a simple blood test to check your iron levels. It is important that your doctor checks both haemoglobin (HB) levels in the blood and ferritin levels in the stores. In runners, HB levels should be 12ng/ml or above and ferritin levels should ideally be 30ng/ml or above.

Make sure that you get an adequate intake of iron from your diet. Red meat is the best source of iron and I always encourage athletes to aim for one portion of lean red meat a week. For vegetarians and vegans, the main tip to remember is to combine vitamin C with plant-based iron-rich foods as vitamin C helps your body to absorb iron. Iron-rich plant foods include:

>>> Fortified cereals

>>> Dark leafy vegetables, such as spinach, kale and broccoli

>>> Lentils and other pulses

Vegetarians can also eat egg yolks for a source of iron.

 Tip *Don't drink tea with your iron-rich foods, or within 30 minutes of eating them, as the phytates in black tea block iron absorption.*

VITAMIN D

Vitamin D is a fat-soluble vitamin that functions as a hormone. Its structure is similar to steroid hormones, such as oestrogen and testosterone. There has been a lot of interest in vitamin D over the last few years. It has always been known for its role in preserving bone health, but it has now also been linked to many other aspects of health, including optimal muscle function.

We make vitamin D in our bodies from sunlight. However, those who live in countries where sunlight might be limited, those who spend little time outdoors, those who cover up with high-factor sunscreen and those who are darker-skinned may actually be at risk of a vitamin-D deficiency. A vitamin-D deficiency can lead to several health issues such as:

>>> Chronic fatigue

>>> Depression

>>> Increased risk of bone injury

>>> Chronic musculoskeletal pain

>>> Viral respiratory tract infections

There also seems to be emerging strong evidence that supplementing an athlete who has sub-optimal levels of vitamin D has real benefits for performance, particularly in strength, power, reaction time, and balance.

There is no universally accepted definition for vitamin-D deficiency, but practitioners use the following guidelines for analyzing blood levels of vitamin D:

>>> Blood levels below 50nmol/l – vitamin-D deficiency

>>> Blood levels below 75nmol/l – insufficient levels of vitamin D

>>> Blood levels between 75 and 120nmol/l – ideal levels of vitamin D

Vitamin-D supplements are readily available, but always make sure that you buy your supplements from a reputable source.

Although you will not be able to meet your requirements through food alone, there are small amounts of vitamin D in certain foods:

>>> Oily fish

>>> Egg yolks

>>> Fortified foods such as milk, margarine and cereals

HAVE YOU LOST YOUR PERFORMANCE MOJO?

We know that good nutrition and regular exercise are essential components of a healthy lifestyle. However, what about when we lose sight of why we started training in the first place? Perhaps it was to drop a few kilos or improve cardiovascular health, or maybe it was a bet that you definitely were not going to lose face over? Regardless of why you started, the fact that you have continued means that you gained something from it: a sense of achievement, a better body composition, or maybe more energy. However, perhaps turning up for the weekly triathlon club swim or taking your place at a sprint or Olympic distance triathlon a few times a year just doesn't feel like enough of a challenge. So you set your sights on something new – getting faster, going further, competing in more extreme places. But what does this mean for your body?

In recent years I have had many an athlete, both recreational and elite, walk into my clinic and tell me that they've just lost their 'mojo'. They keep going out to train but motivation is poor, energy levels are low and if they try to attack a speed session, the engine, the power that was always present, has just disappeared. They come looking for a magic potion, but what they get instead is a prescription for rest and recovery, and ideas on how to boost their immune system.

We seem to be living in a society where no matter what you succeed in, it is never good enough; there is always more you can achieve. We seem to be losing sight of what is actually humanly possible. With the increase in popularity of ultra-endurance events such as Ironman and the rise in the number of events you can take part in all over the world, over a range of distances, we are spoilt for choice. However, this also means we seem to have lost the ability to pace ourselves. I'm lucky enough that I get to work with elite athletes and, in most cases, they choose one or two races a year – these are the ones they focus on. Anything else will be seen as training. Now let's compare this with the recreational athlete. No longer is training for one event a year enough; some individuals are doing them back to back. It never fails to surprise me, when working with someone new, what they have previously completed and what they plan to do next. A typical example is:

>>> End of Feb – 100-mile bike sportive

>>> 2 weeks later – marathon

>>> 3 weeks later – 70.3 Half Ironman

>>> 2 weeks later – Ironman

What surprises me the most, though, is the lack of recovery after each race. It's bad enough that the races are so close together, but many competitors take only one day off before returning to normal training. The elite athletes I work with generally take a minimum of between one and two weeks off post-race and then build back slowly so as not to over-reach the body.

So what does happen when we think the body is invincible and we cause it to over-reach? And how can we overcome this? Over-reaching can have a huge impact on your immune system and it is often this that leads to the loss of your 'mojo'. In order to prevent your body from reaching this point, there are several things I recommend.

GET NUTRITION SMART

Always make sure you tailor your nutrition to your training. If you are going to increase your intensity, distance or number of races, you also need to adjust your intake of carbohydrate and protein so that your body has sufficient fuel to train and recover. I have seen many athletes who cut back on carbs significantly at the same time as they increase their training; they report feeling amazing to start with – and then 6–12 months down the line, their bodies fight back. Carbohydrate, although feared by many, is an essential nutrient for the exercising body. Whilst you should be mindful of portion sizes and the types of carb you're eating, I never advocate a completely ketogenic diet.

BOOST YOUR IMMUNE SYSTEM

Although I always prefer individuals to get their nutrition from their diets, there are a few nutrients that can be difficult to obtain. Both vitamin D (see page 107) and probiotics have a really important function to play in immune health. I recommend a high-dose supplement of vitamin D and probiotic to all my athletes, especially through the winter months.

Hydration is also key for immune function. Saliva is our first line of defence, as it contains IgA. If we are dehydrated, we produce less saliva and in turn this can make us more susceptible to infections and illness.

GET TESTED

If you start to notice that you are lacking energy during training *and* at rest, it is always worth asking your GP to take some blood tests. I usually recommend an athlete is tested for blood levels of iron and ferritin, vitamin D, CRP and thyroid function, as these can indicate if the body is under stress.

SLEEP

The relationship between sleep and sports performance is a huge area of research. What we know already is that it is necessary to have enough good-quality sleep for training recovery and for immune health. Many individuals I have worked with complain about poor sleep and then admit that the last thing they do before they go to bed is check their phone! Increasingly, we are being told how the blue light in phones can disrupt sleep. Switch off your phone at least half an hour before you go to bed – try reading or listening to music instead! Also, be aware that training late in the evening can affect your ability to sleep.

TRAIN SMART AND MONITOR

I'm a big believer in monitoring well-being and performance, and I regularly get athletes to keep a log of the following:

>>> Resting heart rate (although get nocturnal HR data if you can – it's more accurate as there is less room for error with more control over the environment and external factors; less deviation owing to changes in temperature, noise, activity and light)

>>> Sleep quantity and quality

>>> Motivation to train

>>> Energy levels

These measures tell us a lot about how we are feeling. Most sports watches have the ability to monitor heart rate, at rest, during exercise and at night. HR data informs us about what is going on in the body. A resting (nocturnal) HR reading elevated by even just 10 percent from basal levels could indicate illness, fatigue and not sufficient recovery. Take a rest day and ideally wait until HR levels return to normal before training at a high intensity again. Low motivation to train could indicate that you are tired.

OVER-TRAINING AND OVER-REACHING

As triathletes we often push ourselves to improve our performance and meet specific goals. This is not a problem as long as you listen to your body, rest when you need to and fuel appropriately. However, sometimes things can get out of balance; we choose not to rest or recover adequately, which can present itself in many ways, but always ends with poor performance outcomes.

Over-training syndrome, or OTS, can best be defined as the state in which training has repeatedly stressed an athlete's body to the point at which rest is no longer adequate to allow for recovery. It is the name given to a collection of emotional, behavioural and physical symptoms that occur as a result of over-training and have persisted for weeks to months. This is different from the day-to-day variation in performance and post-exercise tiredness that is common in conditioned athletes. Over-training is marked by cumulative exhaustion that persists even after recovery periods and often precedes over-reaching symptoms.

It's not always easy to identify OTS: although the list of symptoms below can guide you, you may not exhibit them all. That said, there are several ways in which you can objectively measure it. One such method includes documenting your heart rate at specific training intensities and speeds over a period of time. If your pace at a given intensity starts to slow, but your heart rate is increased or your resting heart rate increases, or the perceived effort of doing an easy session is consistently higher than it should be, you may be heading into over-reaching. If you ignore the signs of over-reaching, eventually you'll develop full-blown OTS. Some signs and symptoms are:

>>> Lack of energy

>>> Mild leg soreness, general aches and pains

>>> Pain in muscles and joints

>>> Sudden drop in performance

>>> Insomnia

>>> Headaches

>>> Decrease in immunity, leading to more colds and sore throats

>>> Decrease in training capacity/intensity

>>> Moodiness and irritability

>>> Depression/low mood

>>> Lack of motivation to train

>>> Decreased appetite

>>> Increased incidence of injuries

>>> A compulsive need to exercise

>>> An increase in resting heart rate by 10 percent or more

Research into OTS shows that getting adequate rest is the most important thing to overcoming it. Total recovery can take several months, or even years; and some athletes may never fully recover their original athletic form.

Identifying and acting on over-reaching symptoms has a much more positive outcome. Encouraging rest and recovery, reducing stress (both physical and emotional), adopting a nutritious diet of complex carbohydrates, lean protein, and fruits and vegetables, and staying hydrated, will help a runner return to physical form. Try the delicious smoothies and salads in the recipe section to help boost your immune system and provide your body with a nutrient-dense diet.

DISEQUILIBRIUM AND THE POTENTIAL PROBLEMS

Sometimes training and nutrition can become imbalanced. OTS is one example of how the body responds to this imbalance, but there are other potential problems that can occur if good nutrition and good rest do not make up an integral part of your training programme.

When we are training hard, sometimes it is difficult to detect if we are getting sufficient amounts of energy to meet our day-to-day needs, as well as our increased exercise demands. In general terms if you listen to your body, and fuel as required for your chosen activity and intensity, you can maintain your body's equilibrium. However, in some cases, the energy demands of training can be a challenge to meet. For some this will result in weight loss (which may or may not be wanted and which needs to be addressed accordingly). Sometimes, it is not so clear-cut. There are occasions when weight stays stable, but available energy is low; energy intake is not sufficient to meet daily requirements, whether this is owing to a conscious decision to restrict nutritional intake (disequilibrium is sometimes because of an eating disorder) or simply an inability to meet the demands of training. When energy availability is low the body preserves energy by deeming the reproductive system as not essential, therefore lowering the level of sex hormones in the body. This is easy to detect in females as it usually represents itself as a missed period; it is much harder to detect in males. In both genders this situation needs urgent addressing.

Vitamin D and calcium are important for bone health. However, low energy availability can also lead to significant decreases in bone density and overall bone health. In the female athlete, missing three periods consecutively can have potentially negative effects on bone health.

Similarly, body-fat levels that are too low also have a negative effect on bone density. In female athletes, dropping to a body fat of 12 percent or below will once again suppress sex hormones and cause menstruation to cease. In male athletes, a level of 6 percent or below will have a negative effect on bone health, in particular bone density. DEXA scans can be used to measure bone density. A low level is used to diagnose osteoporosis, which is a potentially serious condition that compromises bone strength and may predispose someone to an increased risk of fractures.

By restoring energy availability, it is possible to reverse the effects on bone health in the following ways. Adequate energy availability promotes bone health:

>>> Directly by stimulating the production of hormones that promote bone formation

>>> Indirectly by preserving menstruation and oestrogen production that stems bone resorption

Another variable to consider is a low carbohydrate intake; with the rise in ultra-distance events, more and more individuals are turning to a ketogenic diet – a very low carbohydrate diet where intakes of carbohydrate are no more than 50g a day. As discussed previously, the theory is that in a carbohydrate-depleted state, the body has to use fat as its chosen fuel for all demands, including exercise. This then regulates the use of fat as fuel, potentially making you a more efficient athlete in long-distance events such as Half to Full Ironman. However, as yet, there are no studies looking at the long-term effects on health of such extreme diets. My own observations in clinic tell me that this is not a sustainable practice and while it may be useful to a degree, athletes should be cautious. The ketogenic diet is certainly not something I would advocate any athlete follows for long periods of time. Instead, I prefer to encourage a periodized approach, including carbohydrates around high-intensity training. In fact, we know that low carbohydrate diets will affect oestrogen production and this is another reason female athletes, even if they are normal weight and body fat, may still not menstruate.

Many runners also avoid carbohydrate in an attempt to lose weight. This has become a very common practice as a result of claims in the media from celebrity/health and fitness bloggers, many of whom don't have nutritional qualifications or any scientific understanding of the role of carbohydrate in the body. The only way to lose weight is to take in less energy than you utilize. However, even that requires treading a fine line: increasing the difference between energy in and energy out too much can cause the body to preserve energy reserves and hamper weight loss. Carbohydrates get a bad press as it is so easy to over-consume the wrong types of carbohydrate – think back again to the example of jelly babies versus potatoes (see page 17). If you are a triathlete who wants to lose weight, you do not need to cut out carbohydrates, you just need to reduce them and tailor them to your training.

As mentioned, it is difficult to detect problems in male athletes, but some symptoms to look for in both genders that demonstrate low body-fat levels or poor energy availability include:

>>> Feeling extremes in temperature (hot and cold), owing to low body-fat levels and being unable to regulate heat

>>> Feeling dizzy or disorientated because of low blood glucose

>>> Poor/low libido

>>> Poor concentration

>>> Poor sleep patterns

>>> Recurrent stress fractures

>>> Irritability

>>> Poor recovery between sessions and reduced performance

>>> Withdrawal from social circle and situations

In most cases we can restore equilibrium simply by addressing energy needs and encouraging a minimum of 30Kcals/kg BW of fat-free mass and sufficient carbohydrate. I always encourage individuals who have had an episode of low energy to increase their intake of calcium to 1,600mg a day, which is four servings of dairy, and also take a high-dose vitamin-D supplement (see page 107) to aid the recovery process.

However, sometimes things are not quite this simple. If the individual has developed irregular eating patterns or is suffering from an eating disorder, it can take months to restore equilibrium and involves a multi-disciplinary team approach with a registered dietitian/nutritionist, psychologist, coach (if there is one available), and a GP or other doctor.

THE FEMALE HORMONE CYCLE

The menstrual cycle can have a real influence on a female athlete's energy levels and energy intake. During the follicular phase, day 1 to about day 13, where day 1 is the first day of your period, oestrogen levels are rising and peak just before ovulation (in a 28-day cycle around days 14/15), while progesterone levels are low. During the luteal phase, roughly days 16–28, oestrogen levels decrease, falling to the lowest levels just before your period starts; progesterone is at its highest point midway through this luteal phase. These hormones control what type of fuel you utilize.

It has been well documented that when oestrogen levels are high, that is just before you ovulate, women use a higher percentage of fat for energy. As oestrogen levels drop and progesterone levels rise, our bodies become more dependent on carbohydrate for fuel, which explains the sugar cravings most women experience just before their period. Additionally, high progesterone levels are linked to an increase in protein catabolism, the breakdown of proteins.

These hormone changes also influence temperature change within the body – most women find that a reduction in oestrogen and increase in progesterone during the luteal phase causes a rise in temperature. How many of you that are not near post-menopausal age have woken up with night sweats and wondered what this is about? Now you know! This increase in temperature is also linked to a small increase in overall energy expenditure, which helps to explain the increased hunger and appetite we also tend to feel during this time.

From a nutritional point of view, I suggest that in the 7–10 days prior to your period, so during the luteal phase of your menstrual cycle, you make small dietary changes. Aim to include small frequent snacks of both complex carbohydrate and protein every 2–3 hours to prevent blood-sugar fluctuations. Some good examples include:

>>> Fat-free Greek yogurt with fruit and honey

>>> Hot chocolate made with milk (see Recovery Hot Chocolate, page 197)

>>> Wholegrain toast with Nut Butter (see page 132)

>>> Eggs on toast

>>> Dried fruit and nuts

>>> Oatcakes with cheese

As we have already seen, the levels of hormones during your menstrual cycle can influence the types of fuel you will use for energy. This has a significant impact during ultra-distance events. During such events your body will ultimately run out of glycogen and thus readily available glucose stores within a couple of hours; it will look for other means to provide energy for the working muscles. This could be via fuel you take on during your event – or gluconeogenesis is a further potential pathway for this. Gluconeogenesis is a method by which the body breaks down non-carbohydrate sources of fuel into glucose. The most common of these sources within the body will be fatty acids from fat stores and amino acids from muscle.

However, at certain points of your menstrual cycle – namely just after ovulation and at the start of the luteal phase (that is, when both oestrogen and progesterone levels are equal) – gluconeogenesis is suppressed. This means that in order to continue to meet your fuel requirements for the duration of your ultra-distance event, you will need to take on sufficient amounts of carbohydrate; 90g of carbohydrate per hour has been quoted as the optimal amount needed.

••

A PAIN IN THE GUTS!

A very common and unpleasant side effect most runners will experience at some stage is the phenomenon often known as 'runners trots', that is an urgent need to defecate.

There are a number of reasons why this can occur:

1 > Leaving little time between eating and training; when you start training, in particular running, the body directs blood flow to the working muscles, and away from the digestive system. This combined with the actual physical movement of running causes the contents of the stomach to be thrown up and down, thus leading to that all-too-familiar immediate need to go to the toilet!

2 > Similarly, in longer endurance events, when you are most likely to be using sports gels and drinks, becoming dehydrated and/or taking on more energy than you need causes the contents of the stomach to become very concentrated and this in turn causes stomach issues.

3 > Caffeine is well known for causing an increase in speed of food through the digestive system. This can be advantageous as you can be sure that your digestive system is 'empty' prior to training or competing. Some energy gels and products contain caffeine and while this can have positive effects on your performance, if you are not used to using caffeine with your training, it may cause you some issues, so it best to always practise taking on caffeine in training.

4 > Too much fluid. Some triathletes panic about becoming dehydrated and so aim to take on fluid before and often during their run, even if it is short. Again drinking too much can cause an increase in speed of food through the gut, once again leading to stomach issues.

5 > Change in position; in longer events such as Half to Full Ironman, the change from sitting in a bent over position on the bike for several hours, to suddenly being upright and running can prove problematic. If the change from cycling to running causes you discomfort, I would advise testing different strategies for nutrition and hydration during BRICK sessions.

For most triathletes, addressing these issues can limit problems with having the 'trots' to the occasional bout. However, there is a small percentage of athletes who really struggle with stomach issues, no matter what they do. Even after reducing fluid, training in a fasted state and avoiding high-fibre foods, they still have problems – in some cases, on every session. This obviously can become very distressing and also debilitating, preventing an individual from going out on training sessions because of concerns about getting caught short.

FODMAP DIET

In these cases, something that has been useful to a lot of the athletes I have worked with is following a low FODMAP (fermentable oligosaccharides, disaccharides, monosaccharides and polyols) diet. FODMAPs are short-chain carbohydrates and polyols found in the foods we eat. In some people, the FODMAP molecules are poorly absorbed in the small intestine of the digestive tract, which means they continue their journey along the digestive tract, arriving at the large intestine, where they act as a food source to the bacteria that live there. The bacteria then digest/ferment these FODMAPs and can cause symptoms of irritable bowel syndrome (IBS), including abdominal bloating and distension, excess wind (flatulence), abdominal pain, nausea, changes in bowel habits (diarrhoea, constipation, or a combination of both), and other gastro-intestinal symptoms.

I recommend that you embark on a low FODMAP diet only under the supervision of a fully trained dietitian. It is not a long-term strategy, lasting for a period of only 4–6 weeks, by which time – if FODMAPs are the cause of your symptoms – your symptoms will be significantly improved. If symptoms have not improved, then it is unlikely that FODMAPs are the trigger.

If they do improve, you will enter a re-introduction phase, to help you work out which specific FODMAP food (or foods) is the culprit for your symptoms – sometimes there may be more than one. Often the results are surprising – I have had many runners who have been on a FODMAP diet, convinced that it is gluten or dairy causing their gastro-intestinal symptoms, only to find that it is actually onion and sweetcorn!

It is worth noting here that once again the hormonal affects of the menstrual cycle can have a huge influence on stomach issues. Most women will find that they are most likely to have problems around ovulation and then immediately before their period is due.

BREAKFASTS

Breakfast Shake Serves 1

Preparation time: 5 minutes

This makes a great on-the-go breakfast, or is perfect for recovery after an early-morning training session.

125g/4½oz/½ cup low-fat fruit yogurt, any flavour
200ml/7fl oz/¾ cup skimmed milk

30g/1oz/heaped ¼ cup rolled oats
1 tbsp clear honey

Put all the ingredients in a blender and blend until smooth. Serve straight away.

Nutrition facts (per smoothie)
Calories 344   Carbohydrate 60g   Protein 16g   Fat 3.5g (of which saturates 0g)

Summer Fruit Smoothie Serves 1

Preparation time: 5 minutes

A refreshing pre-workout smoothie full of summer berries, which are known for their vaso-dilation properties, encouraging more oxygen uptake to working muscles.

10 raspberries
5 strawberries
1 tbsp redcurrants

100g/3½oz/⅓ cup fat-free Greek yogurt
1 handful of ice
100ml/3½fl oz/⅓ cup skimmed milk

Put all the ingredients in a blender and blend until smooth. Serve straight away.

Nutrition facts (per smoothie)
Calories 183   Carbohydrate 36g   Protein 10g   Fat 0g (of which saturates 0g)

Mango & Banana Smoothie Serves 1

Preparation time: 5 minutes

This is a refreshing smoothie that is ideal before an early-morning swim session or as a top up prior to a high-intensity training session later on in the day.

100g/3½oz fresh or frozen peeled and pitted mango
1 banana

100g/3½oz/⅓ cup fat-free Greek yogurt
150ml/5fl oz/scant ⅔ cup orange juice

Put all the ingredients in a blender and blend for up to a minute until smooth. Can be kept overnight in a shaker or served immediately.

Nutrition facts (per smoothie)
Calories 308   Carbohydrate 65g   Protein 12.9g   Fat 1g (of which saturates 0g)

The Morning Refresher Smoothie

Serves 1

Preparation time: 5 minutes

Ginger is high in antioxidants, known for its stomach-settling properties and adds real zing to this smoothie, which can be enjoyed at any time of the day.

1 apple, peeled, cored and chopped
1cm/½in piece of root ginger, peeled

100ml/3½fl oz/generous ⅓ cup apple juice
100g/3½oz/⅓ cup lemon-flavoured yogurt

Put all the ingredients in a blender and blend for up to a minute until smooth. Can be kept overnight in a shaker or served immediately.

Nutrition facts (per smoothie)
Calories 243   Carbohydrate 54.5g   Protein 5.6g   Fat 1.7g (of which saturates 0.8g)

Blueberry Bircher Muesli Serves 1

Preparation time: 5 minutes, plus overnight soaking

This is one of my all-time favourite breakfasts, especially in the summer months after an easy early morning run with my spaniel, Bailey. The complex carbohydrate from the oats combined with the high protein from the Greek yogurt mean that this breakfast provides me with slow-release energy all the way through to lunch.

For the Blueberry Compôte
  (makes 4 servings):
350g/12oz/2½ cups blueberries

For the Bircher Muesli:
85g/3oz Blueberry Compôte
30g /1oz/heaped ¼ cup rolled oats
170g/6oz/heaped ⅔ cup fat-free Greek yogurt
2 tsp clear honey

1 Put the blueberries in a saucepan with 4 tablespoons water over a medium heat. Bring to the boil, then turn the heat down to low and simmer for about 10 minutes until the blueberries are soft and slightly thickened.

2 Leave the compôte to cool, then transfer to a screw-topped jar and keep in the fridge for up to 3 days.

3 To make the Muesli, put a quarter of the Blueberry Compôte (85g/3oz) in a bowl, stir in the oats, cover and leave to soak in the fridge overnight.

4 Stir in the yogurt and honey and enjoy.

Nutrition facts (per serving)
Calories 291   Carbohydrate 52.2g   Protein 17.3g   Fat 2.5g (of which saturates 0g)

Toasted Walnut & Honey Porridge

Serves 1

Preparation time: 5 minutes   **Cooking time:** 10 minutes

This porridge is the perfect choice pre- or post-high-intensity training run; walnuts are one of the only plant sources of omega 3 fats. To save time you could toast the walnuts in larger batches and keep them in an airtight container for a few days.

25g/1oz/scant ¼ cup walnuts
50g/1¾oz/½ cup rolled oats

250ml/9fl oz/1 cup skimmed milk
1 tbsp honey

1 Toast the walnuts in a non-stick frying pan for a few minutes until golden and beginning to smell toasted.

2 Put the oats and milk in another saucepan set over a low heat, bring to the boil, simmer for 3–5 minutes, stirring occasionally until the milk has been absorbed by the oats and the porridge/oatmeal is thick.

3 Transfer to a bowl, top with toasted walnuts and swirl over the honey. Serve immediately.

Nutrition facts (per serving)
Calories 498   Carbohydrate 65g   Protein 20g   Fat 18g (of which saturates 1.4g)

HERO FOOD: MILK

It has been well documented that milk is the ideal choice for recovery from high-intensity exercise. When you look at the recommendations for recovery in terms of carbohydrate and protein, the suggested amounts are equal to a 3:1 ratio of carbohydrate to protein. This ratio ensures ideal recovery for the body, particularly after high-intensity exercise, training or competition, when glycogen stores will be completely or close to completely depleted. This is further enhanced if carbohydrate is in a fast release form and protein is easily digestible. The milk sugar (lactose) and whey protein in milk provide this balance, making it a perfect recovery choice. Additionally, milk is a good source of minerals and electrolytes, which are also important for rehydrating post exercise.

Apple Breakfast Bread Makes 8 slices

Preparation time: 10 minutes   **Cooking time:** 30 minutes

There is no longer an excuse to not eat breakfast. Whether you claim to be just 'not a breakfast' person or leave the house very early, this bread is easy to prepare in advance and provides a nutritious breakfast eaten on its own or toasted and topped with honey or Nut Butter (see page 131). It also doubles up as a portable snack to eat either before or during a high-intensity training session.

a little rapeseed/canola oil, for greasing
150g/5½oz/scant 1¼ cups spelt flour
200g/7oz/1⅓ cups wholemeal flour
½ tsp salt
1 tsp bicarbonate of soda/baking soda
1 large or 2 small eating apples, such as
    Cox's, peeled, cored and coarsely grated

55g/2oz/scant ½ cup walnuts, chopped
60ml/2fl oz/¼ cup walnut oil
2 tbsp clear honey
1 egg
200ml/7fl oz/¾ cup apple juice

1 Preheat the oven to 180°C/350°F/Gas 4 and lightly grease a 450g/1lb loaf pan.

2 Mix together the flours, salt and bicarbonate of soda/baking soda in a bowl, then fold in the grated apple. Reserve 1 tablespoon of the nuts, then stir the rest into the mixture. Gently stir in the walnut oil, honey, egg and apple juice, being careful not to over-mix. Spoon the mixture into the prepared pan and scatter the reserved nuts over the top.

3 Bake for 30 minutes, or until a skewer inserted in the centre comes out clean.

4 Leave to cool in the pan for 10–15 minutes, then turn out and transfer to a wire rack. Serve warm or cold. The loaf will keep in an airtight container for up to 3 days.

Nutrition facts (per serving)
Calories 173   Carbohydrate 27.5g   Protein 6g   Fat 5.2g (of which saturates 0g)

Race Day Bagel with Nut Butter Serves 1

Preparation time: 35 minutes **Cooking time:** 3 minutes

Bagels are packed with carbohydrate, ideal for before an endurance event: 60g carbohydrate from one bagel compared with 30–40g from two slices of toast or 50g/1¾oz rolled oats – and this is topped with a banana. The Nut Butter helps to slow down the carb release and prevent blood-sugar dips. You can buy it from the supermarket or health-food store, but making your own from your favourite nuts just takes a little patience. Walnuts are high in omega-3 fats, so make a nutritious butter that is especially good in savoury dishes, mixed with pesto or used in cake recipes that include walnuts. Almonds are high in calcium so are a great choice for vegans or those who struggle to get enough calcium without dairy options. Brazil nuts are high in the antioxidant selenium, which is necessary for many biological processes within the body.

For the Nut Butter (makes 310g/11oz):
310g/11oz/2 cups whole nuts of your choice,
   such as almonds, hazelnuts, cashew nuts
   or walnuts

For the Race Day Bagel:
1 wholemeal bagel
25g/1oz Nut Butter
1 large banana

1 First make the Nut Butter. Put the nuts in a food processor and run the machine for 12–15 minutes, stopping regularly to scrape the nuts down the side of the processor bowl and loosen the mixture from the base. Continue to process until the nuts are finely ground and form a ball around the blade. Keep processing until the nuts release their oil and the mixture forms a soft, smooth butter. Store in an airtight jar in the fridge for up to 3 weeks.

2 Preheat the grill/broiler to high.

3 Slice the bagel in half horizontally and toast the cut sides, then spread them with the Nut Butter. Slice the banana on top and serve straight away.

Nutrition facts (per serving)
Calories 470 Carbohydrate 80g Protein 18g Fat 18g (of which saturates 2g)

English Breakfast Muffins Makes 12

Preparation time: 20 minutes   **Cooking time:** 35 minutes

This is a portable alternative to the classic English breakfast, making it a good choice for when you are on the move or feel the need for a higher-protein option.

a drizzle of olive oil, for frying
6 slices lean bacon
½ small onion, diced
100g/3½oz tomatoes, chopped into chunks
8 large eggs

2 tbsp milk
200g/7oz/3½ cups fresh breadcrumbs
100g/3½oz Cheddar cheese, grated
sea salt and freshly ground black pepper

1 Preheat the oven to 200°C/400°F/Gas 6 and grease a 12-hole muffin pan.

2 Add a drizzle of oil to a large non-stick frying pan and fry the bacon slices for about 5 minutes until cooked and beginning to brown. Remove from the pan and leave until cool enough to handle, then chop into small pieces. Set aside.

3 In the same pan, add another drizzle of oil and fry the onion for 5–10 minutes, or until golden brown. Add the tomatoes and cook until softened, then set aside.

4 Whisk together the eggs and milk and season with a pinch of salt and pepper. Reserve a little of the bacon and cheese for the topping, then stir the remainder into the eggs along with the breadcrumbs, tomato and onion.

5 Spoon the mixture evenly into the muffin pan holes and sprinkle the remaining bacon and cheese over the top. Bake in the preheated oven for 20–25 minutes, or until cooked through.

6 To remove the muffins from the pan, run a small butter knife around the cups to loosen and pull up. Serve warm.

Nutrition facts (per serving)
Calories 264   Carbohydrate 13.4g   Protein 16.4g   Fat 15.7g (of which saturates 5.8g)

Scrambled Egg Pitta Serves 1

Preparation time: 5 minutes   **Cooking time:** 5 minutes

This is a powerhouse of a breakfast. Two large eggs provide around 20g protein, which is the recommended amount to consume in the recovery phase after exercise. When stuffed into a wholemeal pitta, you add some complex carbohydrate, making this an effective recovery meal.

2 large eggs
1 tbsp skimmed milk
1 large wholemeal pitta bread

sea salt and freshly ground black pepper
1 tbsp apple chutney, to serve

1 Put the eggs and milk in a bowl and whisk together until fluffy. Season with a little salt and pepper. Pour into a non-stick saucepan over a low heat and cook for 2–3 minutes, stirring continuously, until the eggs have stiffened and come away from the side of the pan.

2 Meanwhile, heat the grill/broiler to high and toast the pitta bread, then slice it open. Spoon the scrambled egg mixture into the pocket of the pitta and serve hot or cold with a spoonful of chutney.

Nutrition facts (per serving)
Calories 303 Carbohydrate 30g Protein 19g Fat 10.7g (of which saturates 3.3g)

HERO FOOD: EGGS

They may be small, but eggs really pack a punch when it comes to nutritional value; 2 medium eggs will provide you with around 15g of protein, 100 per cent of your daily requirement of vitamin B_{12} (essential for the formation of red blood cells) and are also packed with selenium, a powerful antioxidant. A lot of people still avoid eggs due to the concern over cholesterol, but in fact a medium egg only contains 4.6g of fat, of which only 1.3g comes from saturated fat. Studies have also shown that individuals who consumed two eggs for breakfast every morning ate 300 calories less the rest of the day, making eggs a great start to the day on low intensity or rest days!

Buckwheat Pancakes with Strawberries & Vanilla Yogurt Serves 4

Preparation time: 10 minutes, plus 30 minutes' resting (optional) **Cooking time:** 15 minutes

Using buckwheat for these pancakes makes them a useful wheat-free option, as well as giving the dish the slightly more nutty flavour and texture that I prefer. Buckwheat is also a great source of complex carbohydrate, making these pancakes a perfect choice before a hard training session.

270ml/9½fl oz/generous 1 cup skimmed milk
1 egg
a pinch of sea salt

115g/4oz/scant 1 cup buckwheat flour
3 tbsp rapeseed/canola oil
200g/7oz strawberries, hulled and chopped
400g/14oz/1⅔ cups low-fat vanilla yogurt

1 Put the milk, egg and salt in a large bowl and mix together well.

2 Sift the buckwheat flour into a separate bowl. Gradually add the flour to the milk mixture, stirring constantly until you have a smooth batter. You can make the pancakes straight away or cover the batter and leave to rest in the fridge for 30 minutes.

3 Heat a pancake or frying pan until hot, then add 1 teaspoon of the oil and swirl to coat the base of the pan. Pour in about 3 tablespoons of the pancake mixture and again swirl the pan to spread it evenly over the base. Cook for 1–2 minutes until golden underneath, then flip over and brown the other side. Remove from the pan and keep warm. Continue to fry 7 more pancakes, layering the cooked pancakes with baking paper and keeping them warm while you cook.

4 Put a handful of chopped strawberries and 2 heaped tablespoons vanilla yogurt into the centre of each pancake and fold into a triangle to serve.

Nutrition facts (per serving)
Calories 314   Carbohydrate 34.5g   Protein 13g   Fat 13.9g (of which saturates 2.3g)

Oaty Banana Pancake Serves 1

Preparation time: 5 minutes   **Cooking time:** 8 minutes

Another alternative to the traditional batter pancake, this recipe is relatively fuss-free so is great to make in the morning, even before work. Oats are the main ingredient, they are packed full of slow-release carbohydrate and soluble fibre, ensuring that you not only stay full until lunchtime but you are also less likely to reach for the biscuit barrel or cookie jar mid-afternoon. That also means it gives you plenty of stamina as a pre-training option.

100g/3½oz/1 cup rolled oats
1 egg
1 tbsp low-fat soft cheese

2 tbsp skimmed milk
1 banana, chopped
2 tsp clear honey

1 Put the oats, egg, cream cheese and milk in a bowl and whisk until you have a smooth batter.

2 Heat a non-stick frying pan over a medium heat, then pour in half the batter and cook for 4 minutes, or until the pancake is set around the edge with some bubbles through the centre. Flip it over and cook on the other side until golden and set.

3 Serve with chopped banana and a drizzle of honey.

Nutrition facts (per serving)
Calories 371   Carbohydrate 57g   Protein 17g   Fat 9.2g (of which saturates 1.3g)

LIGHT MEALS

Thai Green Chicken Curry Serves 4

Preparation time: 10 minutes   **Cooking time:** 25 minutes

This is a great dish to come home to after a training session. The chicken provides much-needed protein to help muscles recover and repair, while the spices add essential antioxidants to help prevent further stress on the body. If you are recovering from a high-intensity session, serve the curry with a pitta bread.

1 tbsp oil, for frying
2 garlic cloves, finely chopped
1 bunch of spring onions/scallions, finely chopped
185g/6½oz Thai green curry paste
400g/14oz skinless, boneless chicken breast, diced
400ml/14fl oz/generous 1½ cups coconut milk

100g/3½oz fine green beans
100g/3½oz carrots, cut into batons
200g/7oz spinach leaves
2 large courgettes/zucchini, cut into chunks
juice of ½ lime
1 handful of coriander/cilantro leaves, chopped
1 small red chilli, deseeded and chopped (optional)

1 Heat the oil in a wok or large frying pan over a medium heat, add the garlic and spring onions/scallions and fry for a few minutes until they are golden brown. Add the curry paste and cook for a further 3 minutes, stirring occasionally, or until you can smell their aroma.

2 Add the chicken and stir to coat well with the paste.

3 Add the coconut milk and 400ml/14fl oz/generous 1½ cups water, turn the heat up to high and bring to the boil, then turn the heat down to low and simmer for 10 minutes.

4 Add the remaining vegetables and simmer for 8 minutes, or until the chicken and vegetables are just tender. Add the lime juice, coriander/cilantro and chilli for extra spice, if you like.

5 Serve straight away or leave to cool, put in an airtight container and store in the fridge until needed.

Nutrition facts (per serving)
Calories 347   Carbohydrate 15g   Protein 20g   Fat 25g (of which saturates 15.7g)

Chicken & Quinoa Salad Serves 4

Preparation time: 15 minutes, plus 20 minutes cooling   **Cooking time:** 15 minutes

This salad is a great choice to take to work if you have an evening training session planned, or to cook after a late workout when you don't want to spend ages preparing a meal. Quinoa is a slow-release carbohydrate; additionally it is one of the only grains with a high protein content. I have suggested the use of walnut oil here, which adds a nutty taste but also provides omega-3 fats, which can be useful in preventing fatigue.

150g/5½oz/¾ cup quinoa
1 litre/35fl oz/4 cups chicken stock
400g/14oz skinless, boneless, cooked
   chicken, cut into chunks
150g/5½oz cherry tomatoes
100g/3½oz cucumber, chopped

1 red or green pepper, deseeded and
   chopped
1 tbsp walnut oil
1 avocado
juice of ½ lemon
sea salt and freshly ground black pepper

1 Put the quinoa and stock in a saucepan and bring to the boil over a high heat, then turn the heat down to low and simmer for 12 minutes, or until the quinoa is soft and has absorbed most of the stock. Drain off any remaining stock, put the quinoa in a bowl and leave to cool.

2 Add the chicken, tomatoes, cucumber, pepper and oil, season with salt and pepper and toss together to mix.

3 Peel the avocado, remove the pit and cut the flesh into chunks. Toss with the lemon juice, then gently fold into the salad. Serve straight away or put in an airtight container and chill in the fridge for up to 3 days.

Nutrition facts (per serving)
Calories 408   Carbohydrate 33.5g   Protein 30.5g   Fat 17.6g (of which saturates 3.9g)

Spicy Steak Wraps with Tomato Salsa Serves 2

Preparation time: 10 minutes

Wraps make a great alternative to sandwiches and this one is also a good way to use up leftovers. Although red meat has had a bad press recently, it is still the best source of iron available so should be included in your diet in moderation. By choosing a lean steak, you will take on a great source of protein with minimal saturated fat. The salsa is packed full of lycopene-rich tomatoes and red peppers, not forgetting chilli, which is a potent source of capsaicin, known for its antioxidant and anti-inflammatory properties. Further research also suggests a potential role for capsinoids in weight maintenance and improved body fat composition. Plus there's some evidence that chilli can help eliminate congestion, boost immunity and prevent stomach ulcers.

2 lean beef steaks, each 150g/5½oz
1 red pepper, deseeded and sliced
2 wholemeal tortilla wraps

For the Tomato Salsa:
1 small onion
1 red chilli, deseeded
1 garlic clove
1 beef/beefsteak tomato, chopped
2 tsp balsamic vinegar
1 handful of coriander/cilantro leaves, chopped

1 Preheat the grill/broiler. Grill/broil the steaks for 2–3 minutes on each side, depending on the thickness of the steaks, until they are cooked to your preferred doneness.

2 To make the salsa, put the onion, chilli and garlic in a food processor and whiz until finely chopped, almost paste-like. Add the tomato, vinegar and coriander/cilantro and mix together well.

3 Place a steak in the centre of each wrap and divide the sliced peppers and salsa equally between the wraps. Fold the tortillas to encase the filling. Serve straight away, or wrap in cling film/plastic wrap and serve as a portable meal.

Nutrition facts (per serving)
Calories 403   Carbohydrate 37g   Protein 37.5g   Fat 10g (of which saturates 4.4g)

Salmon Muscle-Recovery Wraps <small>Serves 2</small>

Preparation time: 10 minutes

Once training is over, it is essential to think about muscle recovery. Studies show the optimal time for this is within 2 hours of finishing training, but the earlier the better. It is well documented that omega-3 fats help to reduce inflammation but they can also be beneficial in reducing fatigue, so why not try this wrap specially designed for the purpose? The wholemeal tortilla will help to replenish glycogen stores, while the avocado provides further essential fats, the tomatoes include lycopene and there's vitamin B6 from the lettuce.

200g/7oz grilled or canned salmon, skinned and flaked
2 tbsp plain yogurt
1½ tbsp lime juice

2 wholemeal tortilla wraps
½ avocado, peeled, pitted and sliced
2 large tomatoes, sliced
2 handfuls of shredded lettuce

1 Mix the salmon with the yogurt and lime juice.

2 Divide the salmon mixture equally between the wraps and top each one with half the avocado, tomato and lettuce. Roll and fold each wrap to encase the filling. Serve straight away, or wrap in cling film/plastic wrap for a portable meal.

Nutrition facts (per serving)
Calories 534   Carbohydrate 51.8g   Protein 32.5g   Fat 23.1g (of which saturates 4.6g)

Smoked Mackerel Fishcakes Serves 4

Preparation time: 15 minutes, plus 30 minutes chilling   **Cooking time:** 13 minutes

Smoked Mackerel is a great source of omega-3 fatty acids and vitamin D, making this a superb recovery choice to help repair muscle damage. Serve with pittas for extra carbs after a tough track session or with a large salad for lunch on a steady run day.

450g/1lb sweet potatoes
500g/1lb 2oz smoked mackerel fillets
4–6 spring onions/scallions, finely sliced
1 handful chopped coriander/cilantro leaves

½ tsp chilli/hot pepper flakes
wholemeal bread flour, for dusting
1 tbsp olive oil, for frying

1 Put the sweet potatoes in the microwave and cook for about 6–7 minutes until they are soft and cooked through (alternatively you can bake in the oven at 190°C/375°F/Gas 5 for about 45 minutes, depending on the size of the potatoes). Allow to cool a little, then scrape the flesh out into a mixing bowl and mash it – you will need about 350g/12oz.

2 Flake the mackerel and mix it with the mashed sweet potato. Add spring onions/ scallions, chilli/hot pepper flakes and coriander/cilantro, and mix everything together well. Shape the mixture into 8 patties and chill in the fridge for at least 30 minutes.

3 Dust the patties with flour, shaking off any excess. Heat the oil in a frying pan over a medium heat and lightly fry the patties for about 6 minutes, or until golden brown and cooked through, turning over halfway through cooking. Drain on paper towels and serve.

Nutrition facts (per fishcake)
Calories 282   Carbohydrate 10g   Protein 13.3g   Fat 21.3g (of which saturates 2.9g)

Margherita Frittata Serves 4

Preparation time: 15 minutes   **Cooking time:** 10 minutes

Eggs are fantastic for recovery, a real powerhouse of nutrients. This twist on the traditional Magherita pizza makes this a fantastic higher protein version. Serve with a large green salad for a carb-free lunch; add some sourdough toast for boosting glycogen stores either pre or post long run.

8 eggs
1 tbsp rapeseed/canola oil
1–2 garlic cloves, finely chopped
100g/3½oz mushrooms
2 large fresh tomatoes, sliced

a pinch of dried Italian herbs
100g/3½oz mozzarella cheese, sliced
sea salt and freshly ground black pepper
large green salad, to serve

1 **Whisk the eggs in a large bowl and season with salt and pepper. Leave to one side.**

2 **Heat the oil in a large frying pan over a low heat. Fry the garlic until starting to brown, then add the mushrooms and fry for about 3–5 minutes until soft and tender.**

3 **Preheat the grill/broiler to medium-high.**

4 **Pour the egg mixture into the pan and cook over a medium heat for a few minutes until it looks like it will come away from the sides of the pan. Top with slices of tomato, sprinkle with Italian herbs and then top with mozzarella slices. Remove the pan from the heat and put under the hot grill/broiler for 3 minutes, or until the top is golden. Cut into quarters and serve hot with a large green salad.**

Nutrition facts (per serving)
Calories 250   Carbohydrate 5.9g   Protein 19.8g   Fat 16.9g (of which saturates 5.9g)

Egg Fried Rice with Toasted Cashews Serves 4

Preparation time: 10 minutes   **Cooking time:** 25 minutes

Another great quick and easy-to-prepare recovery meal, you'll love this after a high-intensity training session. It is even quicker if you some leftover cooked long-grain rice, in which case you can start at step 2.

200g/7oz/scant 1 cup brown rice
100g/3½oz/scant 1 cup cashew nuts
1 tbsp rapeseed/canola oil
2 garlic cloves, finely chopped
1 large carrot, thinly sliced
100g/3½oz/¾ cup frozen sweetcorn/corn kernels

100g/3½oz/¾ cup frozen peas
3 eggs, lightly beaten
2 tsp soy sauce
1 tbsp chopped coriander/cilantro leaves
freshly ground black pepper

1 Put the rice in a saucepan and cover with cold water. Bring to the boil over a high heat, then partially cover, turn the heat down to low and simmer for 14 minutes, or until the rice is just tender but still has a little bite. Drain and rinse in cold water, then leave in a colander to drain and cool.

2 Meanwhile, put the cashews in a dry frying pan over a medium heat and toss for a few minutes until just beginning to brown. Tip out and leave to one side.

3 Heat the oil in a large frying pan over a medium heat, add the garlic and fry for 3 minutes, stirring gently, or until golden in colour. Add the carrot, sweetcorn/corn and peas and cook for 2–3 minutes, stirring occasionally, until well mixed. Stir in the cooked rice.

4 Turn the heat down to low and slowly stir in the eggs so that they mix with the rice and vegetables and cook through. Add the soy sauce, season with pepper to taste, sprinkle with most of the toasted nuts and coriander and stir them into the rice. Spoon into individual serving bowls, sprinkle with the remaining nuts and coriander/cilantro and serve hot.

Nutrition facts (per serving)
Calories 460   Carbohydrate 56.5g   Protein 14.4g   Fat 20.4g (of which saturates 3.4g)

Miso Noodle Soup Serves 1

Preparation time: 5 minutes   **Cooking time:** 8 minutes

This is so quick and easy to produce, it literally takes minutes and makes a great option to help warm you up after a late night training session or a wet lunch time session! The miso paste helps to replace lost salts, while the noodles and edamame beans provide both carbs and protein, essential for the recovery process.

1 x sachet miso soup paste
1 x 75g/2½oz nest egg noodles

100g/3½oz frozen mixed vegetables
150g/5½oz frozen edamame beans

1 **Put the miso paste, noodles, mixed vegetables and edamame beans in a saucepan.**

2 **Boil the kettle and add 400ml/14fl oz/1¾ cups boiling water to the pan.**

3 **Stir over a low heat for 3–5 minutes, until the noodles and frozen vegetables are tender and cooked through. Spoon into a bowl and serve steaming hot.**

Nutrition facts (per serving)
Calories 490   Carbohydrate 57.4g   Protein 32.8g   Fat 13.8g (of which saturates 4.7g)

Chickpea & Kale Broth Serves 4

Preparation time: 10 minutes   **Cooking time:** 1 hour

Kale is a nutrient-dense vegetable, high in vitamins A and K and – most importantly for sportspeople – a great source of nitrate. The body turns nitrate into nitric oxide, which has been linked to an increased uptake of oxygen into the muscles. Combined with chickpeas and sweet potato, which both help release energy at a slower rate, this dish is tailor-made for pre-training.

1 tbsp rapeseed/canola oil
1 tsp cumin seeds
1 large onion, chopped
2 garlic cloves, crushed
1cm/½in piece of root ginger, peeled and
    finely chopped
1 large sweet potato (about 300g/10½oz),
    chopped

1 red chilli, deseeded and chopped (optional)
1 litre/35fl oz/4 cups vegetable stock
1 large bunch of curly kale, washed and
    torn into smaller pieces
800g/1lb 12oz canned chickpeas, drained
    and rinsed

1 Heat the oil in a large saucepan over a medium heat. Add the cumin seeds and shake the pan for a minute or so until you can smell their aroma. Add the onion, garlic and ginger and fry for 4– 5 minutes, stirring occasionally, until golden brown.

2 Add the sweet potato and chilli, if using, and cook for a further 5 minutes.

3 Pour in the stock and bring to the boil, then turn the heat down to low and simmer for 15–20 minutes until the sweet potato is tender.

4 Add the kale and simmer for a further 20 minutes. Add the chickpeas and simmer for 5 more minutes, stirring occasionally, or until everything is heated through and well blended. Serve hot.

Nutrition facts (per serving)
Calories 294   Carbohydrate 47.9g   Protein 14.4g   Fat 5.9g (of which saturates 0.5g)

Sweet Potato & Red Lentil Soup Serves 4

Preparation time: 10 minutes   **Cooking time:** 35 minutes

Packed full of slow-release carbohydrate and iron-rich lentils, this soup is the perfect lunch choice after a really tough morning training session out in the cold and wet.

1 tbsp rapeseed/canola oil
1 red onion, chopped
1 garlic clove, crushed
4 sweet potatoes (about 1.2kg/2lb 12oz total
   weight) peeled and chopped
85g/3oz/⅓ cup red lentils

1 litre/35fl oz/4 cups vegetable stock
½ tsp paprika
½ tsp ground cumin
½ tsp chilli powder
1 handful of coriander/cilantro leaves,
   chopped

1 Heat the oil in a large saucepan over a medium heat. Add the onion and garlic and cook for 2–3 minutes until tender. Add the sweet potatoes and red lentils and cook for 2 minutes.

2 Add the stock, paprika, cumin and chilli powder, bring to the boil, then turn the heat down to low and simmer for 30 minutes, or until the sweet potatoes are tender and the lentils are cooked.

3 Blend using a hand-held blender or transfer to a blender or food processor and whiz until smooth. Sprinkle with the coriander/cilantro and serve hot.

Nutrition facts (per serving)
Calories 384   Carbohydrate 76g   Protein 12.2g   Fat 3.9g (of which saturates 0.6g)

HERO FOOD: HERBS & SPICES

Herbs and spices are a great way to make even the most basic dish a little more interesting; who wouldn't prefer rosemary infused baked potato wedges over just potato wedges? Or how about the warming properties of ginger when blended with butternut squash for a hearty soup; and you really can't beat the blend of lime, chilli and coriander to add zest and flavour to a stir fry. However it is not just their ability to perk up meals that makes them so important to our daily diets. They are actually very potent and powerful antioxidants and a great way to ensure your immune system gets a boost.

Three-Lentil Dhal with Coriander & Chilli Serves 4

Preparation time: 10 minutes   **Cooking time:** 50 minutes

This recipe is inspired by my mum. She is a fantastic cook and makes the best dhal I have ever tasted! I have added a slight twist to her traditional Punjabi recipe with the addition of some coconut milk and by cooking all the spices together at the start. Lentils are often overlooked but they are cheap, very easy to cook and extremely high in soluble fibre, making them a great choice if you are trying to cut calories as they keep you full for ages.

1 tbsp rapeseed/canola oil
1 tsp cumin seeds
2 garlic cloves, crushed
7cm/2¾in piece of root ginger, peeled and
   finely chopped
1 red chilli, deseeded and chopped
400g/14oz canned chopped tomatoes

1 tsp sea salt
85g/3oz/⅓ cup red lentils
85g/3oz/⅓ cup yellow lentils
85g/3oz/scant ½ cup green lentils
1 handful of coriander/cilantro leaves,
   chopped
2 tbsp coconut cream

1 Heat the oil in a large saucepan over a medium heat. Add the cumin seeds and shake the pan for a minute or so until you can smell their aroma. Add the garlic, ginger and chilli and fry for about 5 minutes, stirring occasionally, until golden brown.

2 Add the tomatoes and salt, stir well and cook for a further 3 minutes. Stir in all the lentils so they are coated in the tomato mixture, then add 750ml/26fl oz/ 3 cups boiling water. Turn the heat down to low and simmer for 30–40 minutes until the lentils have soaked up the water and are tender.

3 Sprinkle with coriander/cilantro, top with a dollop of coconut cream and serve hot.

Nutrition facts (per serving)
Calories 313   Carbohydrate 38g   Protein 13.6g   Fat 12g (of which saturates 3g)

Super Beans on Toast Serves 2

Preparation time: 5 minutes   **Cooking time:** 5 minutes

This was an experimental dish I first made a while back when the cupboards were bare but I needed to put together a quick, light dinner after travelling all day! The yeast extract is optional and can be substituted with soy sauce or even balsamic vinegar if you're not a fan.

400g/14oz canned baked beans
400g/14oz canned kidney beans, drained
   and rinsed
1 tsp yeast extract (optional)

4 slices of wholemeal or rye bread toast
butter or margarine, for spreading
mixed salad, to serve

1 **Heat the baked beans in a saucepan over a medium heat. Stir in the kidney beans and yeast extract until combined and warmed through.**

2 **Toast the bread, then spread with butter or margarine.**

3 **Divide the toast between two serving plates, pour over the bean mixture and serve with a mixed salad.**

Nutrition facts (per serving)
Calories 410   Carbohydrate 59g   Protein 18g   Fat 11g (of which saturates 5g)

Avocado & Feta Toasts Serves 2

Preparation time: 10 minutes   **Cooking time:** 4 minutes

One of my favourite lunches – it was my good friend and talented runner Holly Rush who introduced me to the combination of avocado, feta cheese, lime and chilli flakes.

4 slices seeded bread
1 large avocado, peeled, pitted and
    roughly chopped

60g/2¼oz feta cheese, crumbled
juice of ½ lemon
a pinch of dried chilli/hot pepper flakes

1 **Toast the bread.**

2 **While the bread is toasting, put the avocado, feta, lemon juice and chilli/hot pepper flakes in a bowl and mash together.**

3 **Top the toast with the avocado and cheese mixture and serve immediately.**

Nutrition facts (per serving)
Calories 444   Carbohydrate 37.9g   Protein 14.1g   Fat 29g (of which saturates 8.6g)

HERO FOOD: AVOCADO

Avocados are probably one of the most under-rated fruits, feared by many due to their high fat and energy content. However, the reality is that they are packed full of those very helpful good fats essential for absorbing fat-soluble vitamins such as vitamins A, D, E and K, and are also a great source of vitamin E itself. So, while a 100g/3½oz serving of avocado provides 160 calories and 15g of fat, only 2g of fat is saturated. The fat content makes it a satisfying choice for those watching their weight. Try it as a snack drizzled with balsamic vinegar, or mashed with some lime, chilli/hot pepper flakes and coriander/cilantro as a topping for toast.

Roasted Butternut, Tofu & Sprouted Shoot Salad Serves 4

Preparation time: 20 minutes **Cooking time:** 1 hour

This recipe came about as I had a glut of butternut squash being delivered in my weekly veggie box – I wanted an alternative to soup! The beauty of this recipe is that you can roast the squash whole in the oven and then keep the cooked flesh refrigerated for a couple of days until you are ready to use – although I like to keep it slightly warm for an autumnal salad. Tofu is a great choice of protein for vegetarians and vegans, but can of course be enjoyed by all! The spouted shoots add crunch and antioxidants to this already nutrient-dense meal.

1 large butternut squash
100g/3½oz mini pickled beetroot
150g/3½oz mixed salad leaves
200g/7oz smoked tofu
an 8cm/3¼in piece cucumber, diced

150g/3½oz/1 cup cherry tomatoes
1 large carrot, grated
100g/3½oz mixed sprouting shoots
balsamic vinegar and walnut oil,
   to serve

1 Preheat the oven to 180°C/350°F/Gas 4. Put the squash on a baking sheet and bake whole for about 1 hour, until tender and cooked through. Leave to cool.

2 Scoop the squash flesh out of the skin and roughly chop.

3 Toss all the other ingredients together in a large salad bowl. Add the roasted squash and dress the salad with balsamic vinegar and walnut oil, to taste.

Nutrition facts (per serving without dressing)
Calories 389 Carbohydrate 59.1 Protein 22.4g Fat 8.6g (of which saturates 1.3g)

Beetroot, Feta & Potato Salad Serves 4

Preparation time: 15 minutes **Cooking time:** 1 hour

A great light supper after training, with a good dairy source of protein.

2 baking potatoes, scrubbed

100g/3½oz mini pickled beetroot/beets, drained

150g/5½oz mixed salad leaves

200g/7oz/1⅔ cups cubed feta cheese

50g/1¾oz cucumber, cubed

150g/5½oz/1 cup cherry tomatoes

1 large carrot, sliced

85g/3oz/scant 1 cup green olives with chilli (optional)

1 handful of coriander/cilantro leaves, chopped

balsamic vinegar, to serve

walnut oil, to serve

1 Preheat the oven to 200°C/400°F/Gas 6. Pierce the potatoes with a fork, then bake for 1 hour, or until soft on the inside with a lovely crisp skin. Meanwhile combine all the other salad ingredients in a large salad bowl.

2 Remove the potatoes from the oven. Leave to cool for 10 minutes, then cut into chunks and add to the salad. Toss all the ingredients together. Serve with the vinegar and oil on the side so everyone can add their own.

Nutrition facts (per serving without dressing)
Calories 286   Carbohydrate 35g   Protein 11.2g   Fat 12.4g (of which saturates 7.7g)

HERO FOOD: BEETROOT/ BEETS

In recent years, there has been much hype about the use of beetroot as a performance aid. Studies have demonstrated that the high nitrate content of beetroot encourages oxygen uptake by up to 16 per cent, thus preventing the build-up of acidity and improving performance at high intensities. Studies conclude that a daily consumption of 5mmol of nitrate 1–3 hours before training, prior to competing in events lasting 3–36 minutes are required for this desired performance effect. One main issue is that the nitrate content within beetroot differs, making it difficult to determine how much to eat to meet this 5mmol requirement. Specific beetroot shots/juices have been developed with this in mind, but they are an acquired taste!

Roasted Vegetable & Mozzarella Bruschetta Serves 4

Preparation time: 5 minutes   **Cooking time:** 15 minutes

This is a Mediterranean twist on the humble cheese on toast. It's easy and quick, plus it provides you with the benefits of vegetables rich in antioxidants. Sourdough makes exceptionally good and crisp toast and adds to the overall flavour of this light meal.

2 courgettes/zucchini, sliced
2 red peppers, deseeded and cut into chunks
1 aubergine/eggplant, sliced
100g/3½oz mushrooms, sliced
4 garlic cloves, finely chopped

1 tbsp dried oregano
3 tbsp rapeseed/canola oil
8 slices of sourdough bread
200g/7oz mozzarella cheese, sliced
freshly ground black pepper

1 **Preheat the grill/broiler to medium.**

2 **Put all the vegetables and the garlic on a grill tray, sprinkle with the oregano and drizzle the oil over the top. Toss together so all the vegetables are lightly coated. Grill/broil for 8–10 minutes, turning the vegetables occasionally, until they are soft and golden.**

3 **Toast the bread.**

4 **Spoon the vegetables onto the slices of toast and cover with slices of mozzarella. Put back under the grill/broiler for 5 minutes, or until the cheese has melted. Season with black pepper and serve hot.**

Nutrition facts (per serving)
Calories 459   Carbohydrate 45.7g   Protein 24.5g   Fat 21.1g (of which saturates 6.5g)

Roasted Aubergine, Chickpea and Hummus Wrap Serves 2

Preparation time: 10 minutes   **Cooking time:** 20 minutes

This is another great portable meal, the combination of wholemeal tortilla, chickpeas and hummus make it an ideal option for slow-release carbohydrate to fuel a high-intensity session later in the day, or even en route to a competition.

1 aubergine/eggplant
100g/3½oz hummus
2 wholemeal tortilla wraps

125g/4½oz canned chickpeas, drained
and rinsed

1 Preheat the oven to 200°C/400°F/Gas 6.

2 Pierce the aubergine/eggplant in several places with a fork and bake in the preheated oven for 15–20 minutes until the skin is crispy and the flesh has cooked through – it will have pulled away from the skin and be a soft pulp. Leave to cool.

3 Spoon the aubergine/eggplant flesh from the skin and put it into a small mixing bowl. Add the hummus and mix together well.

4 Divide the hummus mixture between the tortilla wraps and top each wrap with half the chickpeas.

5 Roll or fold up and eat straight away, or wrap in cling film/plastic wrap and keep in the fridge until later.

Nutrition facts (per wrap)
Calories 462   Carbohydrate 65.6g   Protein 18g   Fat 14.4g (of which saturates 1.8g)

Root Vegetable Chips with Dippy Eggs Serves 4

Preparation time: 10 minutes **Cooking time:** 45 minutes

This is a real favourite and it demonstrates how training food can include the whole family. It is also what I call a very low-maintenance meal as it is all cooked in one baking pan – which means less washing up, too! If you are serving this as a recovery meal, then make sure you have two eggs to get your 20g of recovery protein.

1 large floury potato, such as Maris Piper, cut into long strips
1 large sweet potato, cut into long strips
2 parsnips, peeled and cut into long strips
2 large carrots, cut into long strips

2 tbsp rapeseed/canola oil
2 tsp dried rosemary
2 tsp clear honey
4 eggs

1 Preheat the oven to 180°C/350°F/Gas 4.

2 Put all the vegetables in a large baking pan. Mix together the oil, rosemary and honey, then pour the mixture over the vegetables and stir well to coat.

3 Cook for about 40 minutes until the vegetables are almost tender.

4 Remove the baking pan from the oven and make 4 spaces among the vegetables. Crack an egg into each space and return the pan to the oven for about 2–3 minutes until the whites of the eggs have turned opaque but the yolks are still runny. Serve straight away.

Nutrition facts (per serving)
Calories 215   Carbohydrate 30g   Protein 8.3g   Fat 11.6g (of which saturates 1.6g)

MAIN MEALS

One-Pot Chicken Casserole Serves 4

Preparation time: 15 minutes   **Cooking time:** 1 hour

When you are juggling training with a job and perhaps a family, main meals must not only meet your training requirements but also suit your lifestyle. This is a great recipe as the complete meal is made in one pot – plus you can even prepare it the night before and have it ready in the fridge to pop into the oven when you get in from work or training. It's also a good one for your slow cooker, if you have one. An ideal recovery choice, it is full of lean protein and carbohydrate to replace glycogen stores.

4 skinless, boneless chicken breasts
1 large onion, cut into chunks 4 large
   carrots, cut into chunks
2 large parsnips, peeled and cut into chunks
2 baking potatoes, such as Maris Piper,
   peeled and cut into chunks

2 garlic cloves, crushed
juice of 1 orange
1 tbsp clear honey
1 handful of rosemary leaves
1 litre/35fl oz/4 cups chicken stock
sea salt and freshly groundblack pepper

1 Preheat the oven to 180°C/350°F/Gas 4.

2 Put the chicken breasts into a large casserole dish and surround with the onion, carrots, parsnips and potatoes. Mix together the garlic, orange juice, honey and rosemary and stir into the dish. Finally, pour the stock over the chicken and vegetables and season with salt and pepper.

3 Cover and cook for 45–60 minutes until the vegetables are all cooked through and the chicken juices run clear when pierced with a sharp knife. Serve hot.

Nutrition facts (per serving)
Calories 386   Carbohydrate 54.8g   Protein 32.4g   Fat 5.3g (of which saturates 1.9g)

Mustard-Mash Chicken Pie Serves 4

Preparation time: 15 minutes **Cooking time:** 1¼ hours

I associate mashed potato with comfort food but it can be a training food with a few adjustments. By replacing the usual high-fat butter and cheese with cream cheese and mustard, you get a lower-fat alternative that's equally flavoursome. The potato skin is nutritious and adds a delicious crunch. Serve this easy one-pot meal to family or friends and they'd never know that you were following a specific nutrition plan.

1 tbsp rapeseed/canola oil

4 skinless, boneless chicken breasts, cut into chunks

1 onion, chopped

2 carrots, diced

2 courgettes/zucchini, diced

100g/3½oz runner beans, cut into strips

100g/3½oz/¾ cup fresh, podded, or frozen peas

455ml/16fl oz/scant 2 cups chicken stock

sea salt and freshly ground black pepper

For the Mustard Mash:

750g/1lb 10oz floury potatoes, such as Maris Piper, unpeeled, cut into chunks

30g/1oz low-fat cream cheese

1 tsp wholegrain mustard

2–4 tbsp skimmed milk

1 Preheat the oven to 180°C/350°F/Gas 4.

2 Heat the oil in a frying pan over a low heat, add the chicken and onion and fry for about 5 minutes, stirring occasionally, until brown on all sides.

3 Use a slotted spoon to transfer the chicken and onion to a casserole dish. Add the other vegetables, stock, salt and pepper. Cover and bake for 35–40 minutes until the vegetables are tender and the sauce has thickened.

4 Meanwhile, prepare the mash. Put the potatoes in a large saucepan and cover with water. Cover and bring to the boil over a high heat, then turn the heat down to low and simmer for 10 minutes, or until tender. Drain well, then return to the pan. Add the cream cheese, mustard and enough milk to mash to a smooth mash.

5 Remove the casserole lid and pile the mash on top of the chicken and vegetables, then return the dish to the oven for a further 15–20 minutes until the topping is browned and crisp. Serve hot.

Nutrition facts (per serving)
Calories 408   Carbohydrate 44g   Protein 34g   Fat 10.9g (of which saturates 4.1g)

Tangy Chicken Stir-Fry Serves 4

Preparation time: 15 minutes   **Cooking time:** 20 minutes

A stir-fry is one of the easiest, most versatile and nutritious ways of cooking food. Choose your protein – whether it's tofu, beans, fish or chicken – pick a variety of vegetables, herbs and spices and away you go. Serve with noodles or rice for a well-balanced training meal any evening of the week.

250g/9oz dried thin egg noodles
1½ tbsp rapeseed/canola oil
500g/1lb 2oz skinless, boneless chicken
   breast, cut into thin strips
2 tsp grated ginger
2 garlic cloves, crushed
1 small onion, chopped
1 red pepper, deseeded and thinly sliced
150g/5oz mangetout/snow peas or sugar
   snap peas

1 large carrot cut into thin strips
1 large courgette/zucchini, cut into
   thin strips
150g/5oz baby corn
juice of 1 lime
2 tbsp sweet chilli sauce
1 tbsp soy sauce
80ml/2½fl oz/⅓ cup chicken stock
1 handful of coriander/cilantro
   leaves, chopped

1 Cook the noodles in a large saucepan of boiling water for 5 minutes, or until tender. Drain well, then toss with ½ tablespoon of the oil to prevent them sticking together. Leave to one side.

2 Heat the remaining oil in a non-stick wok or large frying pan over a high heat. Add about half the chicken so the wok is not overcrowded, and fry for 2–3 minutes, stirring, until browned. Using a slotted spoon, remove the chicken from the wok and cook the remaining chicken, then remove it from the wok.

3 Add the ginger, garlic and onion to the wok and stir-fry for 2 minutes, or until soft. Add the remaining vegetables and stir-fry for 3 minutes, or until tender but still crisp.

4 Add the lime juice, chilli and soy sauces and stock and bring to the boil. Add the noodles and toss to warm through. Return the chicken to the pan and reheat thoroughly. Sprinkle with the coriander/cilantro and serve hot.

Nutrition facts (per serving)
Calories 515   Carbohydrate 40g   Protein 34.2g   Fat 25.1g (of which saturates 5.7g)

Nepalese Chicken with Rice Serves 4

Preparation time: 10 minutes, plus 30 minutes' marinating   **Cooking time:** 45 minutes

This recipe was inspired by a trip to Nepal when I ran the Manaslu trail race. The taste is superb – plus it is rich in lean protein and high in antioxidants.

1 tsp turmeric
a pinch of sea salt
1 tsp freshly ground black pepper
3 skinless chicken breasts, cubed
1 tsp mustard seeds
1 tsp fenugreek seeds
2 tbsp rapeseed/canola oil
2 garlic cloves, crushed
1 tbsp grated root ginger

2 dried red chillies, deseeded and
   finely chopped
1 tsp ground cumin
2 bay leaves
1 large onion, chopped·
500ml/17fl oz/2 cups chicken stock
2 large tomatoes, chopped
150g/5½oz/¾ cup basmati rice
1 handful of coriander/cilantro
   leaves, chopped

1 Rub the turmeric, salt and pepper all over the chicken, cover and leave to marinate in the fridge for 30 minutes.

2 Put the mustard seeds in a frying pan over a medium heat and dry-roast for a few seconds, or until you can smell their aroma, being careful not to burn the spices, then tip them into a mortar or coffee grinder. Repeat with the fenugreek seeds. Crush to a coarse powder.

3 Heat the oil in a wok over a medium-high heat. Add the spice mixture, garlic, ginger, chillies, cumin and bay leaves and stir-fry for 20 seconds. Add the onion and sauté for 3–6 minutes until slightly translucent. Add the marinated chicken and stir-fry for 4 minutes, then add the stock and tomatoes. Bring to the boil, then turn the heat down to low and simmer for 35 minutes, or until the chicken is tender and the sauce has thickened.

4 Meanwhile, cook the rice in boiling water for 10 minutes, or until tender. Sprinkle the chicken with the coriander/cilantro and serve with the rice.

Nutrition facts (per serving)
Calories 443   Carbohydrate 37.4g   Protein 36g   Fat 15.6g (of which saturates 3.7g)

Char-Grilled Chicken Pasta Salad

Serves 4

Preparation time: 15 minutes   **Cooking time:** 15 minutes

After a hard workout on a long summer day, what better way to refuel than with this pasta salad? It is packed full of the slow-release carbohydrate and lean protein you need. Play around with the salad ingredients and come up with your own favourite combination.

320g/11¼oz/3½ cups wholegrain pasta
1½ tbsp rapeseed/canola oil
150g/5oz fine green beans, halved
500g/1lb 2oz skinless, boneless chicken
 breasts, cut into chunks
10cm/4in piece of cucumber, chopped

150g/5oz/heaped 1 cup sweetcorn/corn
 kernels, frozen or canned with no added
 salt and sugar
150g/5oz/1 cup cherry tomatoes, halved
3 tbsp fat-free plain yogurt
juice of ½ lemon
1 handful of chives, chopped

1 Cook the pasta in a large saucepan of boiling water for 8 minutes, or until tender. Drain well, then toss with ½ tablespoon of the oil to prevent the shapes sticking together. Leave to one side.

2 Meanwhile, cook the beans in a small saucepan of boiling water for 4 minutes, or until tender. Drain well and leave to one side.

3 Heat the oil in a griddle pan, add the chicken and fry for about 5 minutes, stirring occasionally, until cooked through. Leave to one side.

4 Mix the cucumber, sweetcorn/corn, tomatoes and green beans in a large salad bowl. Add the chicken and pasta and toss together gently.

5 Put the yogurt in a small bowl and mix in the lemon juice and chives. Add to the chicken salad and toss once more so that the yogurt dressing has mixed through. Serve straight away or cover with cling film/plastic wrap and keep in the fridge until ready to eat.

Nutrition facts (per serving)
Calories 642   Carbohydrate 66.6g   Protein 38g   Fat 25.3g (of which saturates 5.6g)

Turkey Pesto Kievs Serves 4

Preparation time: 15 minutes **Cooking time:** 30 minutes

To make a change from chicken, this dish uses turkey as a lean protein source. It is also a healthier take on the traditional breaded chicken Kiev that can be bought in the shops. You can use shop-bought pesto but you might like to make your own from my recipe.

4 skinless, boneless turkey fillets
50g/1¾oz Mixed Nut Pesto (see page 181)
2 tsp clear honey

1 tsp rapeseed/canola oil
Roasted Mediterranean Vegetables
   (see page 181), to serve

1 Preheat the oven to 180°C/350°F/Gas 4.

2 Take each turkey fillet and make a slit lengthways, leaving one side uncut. Spread a quarter of the pesto inside each turkey fillet.

3 Mix together the honey and oil in a small bowl, then brush each fillet with the mixture. Bake for 25–30 minutes until the turkey is cooked and the juices run clear when pierced with the tip of a sharp knife. If the top starts to brown too quickly, cover with kitchen foil.

4 Serve with the roasted vegetables.

Nutrition facts (per kiev)
Calories 225   Carbohydrate 3.7g   Protein 28g   Fat 10.7g (of which saturates 2.8g)

Black-Eyed Bean and Chilli Beef Burritos Serves 4

Preparation time: 20 minutes   **Cooking time:** 30 minutes

Eating red meat once a week helps athletes to meet their iron requirements.

1 tbsp olive oil, plus extra for greasing
1 small onion, finely chopped
1 garlic clove, crushed
500g/1lb 2oz lean minced/ground beef
1 tsp ground cumin
1 tsp smoked paprika
¼ tsp chilli powder
400g/14oz can chopped tomatoes
1 red pepper, deseeded and chopped
1 green pepper, deseeded and chopped
2 tablespoons tomato purée/paste

400g/14oz can black-eyed beans, drained
  and rinsed
3 large handfuls of coriander/cilantro
  leaves, chopped
8 wholemeal tortillas
salad leaves, to serve

For the Avocado Dip:
1 ripe avocado
200g/7oz/¾ cup crème fraîche
juice of 1 lime

1 Preheat the oven to 200°C/400°F/Gas 6. Heat the oil in a large frying pan over a medium-high heat. Add the onion and garlic and cook, stirring occasionally, for 5 minutes, or until the onion is tender. Add the beef and cook, stirring, for another 3 minutes, or until the beef is browned.

2 Add the cumin, paprika and chilli powder to the pan and cook, stirring, for 1 minute until aromatic, then add the tomatoes, peppers and tomato purée/paste. Bring the mixture to the boil, then reduce heat to medium-low and simmer, uncovered, for 10 minutes until the sauce has thickened. Stir in the beans and coriander/cilantro.

3 Warm the tortillas, following the packet instructions. Divide the beef among the tortillas, spreading it along the centre, and roll up to enclose the filling. Place the burritos in a greased baking dish and bake for 10 minutes until they start to brown.

4 Meanwhile, make the avocado dip. Mash the avocado in a small bowl. Add the crème fraîche and lime juice and mix until well combined. Serve the burritos with the avocado dip and salad leaves.

Nutrition facts (per 2-burrito serving)
Calories 665   Carbohydrate 51.5g   Protein 38.9g   Fat 32.4g (of which saturates 12g)

Sausage Casserole Serves 4

Preparation time: 15 minutes   **Cooking time:** 1 hour

Although we should be reducing our overall intake of processed meat, including it occasionally is not a problem. Choose good-quality sausages – there is a huge range – or another option is you could, like me, use tofu-based sausages instead. I do like one-pot meals that can just be put in a slow cooker or in the oven and left to cook while you get on with other things. This meal is also a sneaky way of getting reluctant vegetable eaters to eat some veggies!

8 lean sausages
400g/14oz canned chopped tomatoes
400g/14oz canned baked beans
1 large courgette/zucchini, cut into chunks
2 large carrots, cut into chunks
2 garlic cloves, finely chopped

4cm/1½in piece of root ginger, peeled
   and finely chopped
150g/5½oz fine green beans, halved
1 tsp paprika
1 handful of rosemary leaves
wholegrain toast, to serve

1 Preheat the oven to 180°C/350°F/Gas 4.

2 Put all the ingredients except the toast in a casserole dish and stir well.
   Cover and cook for about 1 hour until the sausages and vegetables are cooked.

3 Serve with wholegrain toast.

Nutrition facts (per serving)
Calories 309   Carbohydrate 36.3g   Protein 22.7g   Fat 9.1g (of which saturates 2.7g)

Chilli Chard & Pork Rice Serves 4

Preparation time: 15 minutes **Cooking time:** 20 minutes

This dish came about because we get a vegetable box delivered from a local farm and, during spring, there always seems to be an abundance of chard! Chard is very similar to spinach so is also high in folate, iron and nitrates.

1 tbsp rapeseed/canola oil
1 onion, thinly sliced
3 garlic cloves, finely chopped
500g/1lb 2oz pork fillets, cut into strips
120g/4¼oz/heaped ½ cup basmati rice

175g/6oz chard
1 small red chilli, deseeded and finely
  chopped
juice of 1 lemon
sea salt and freshly ground black pepper

1 Heat the oil in a large saucepan over a medium heat, add the onion and garlic and fry for about 4 minutes, stirring occasionally, until golden.

2 Add the pork strips and cook over a low heat for about 5 minutes until they are browned and tender.

3 Add the rice, chard, chilli and lemon juice to the pan, then pour in 500ml/17fl oz/ 2 cups water and season with salt and pepper. Bring to the boil over a high heat, then turn the heat down to low and simmer for about 8 minutes, stirring occasionally, until all the water has been absorbed.

4 Serve hot or leave to cool and serve cold.

Nutrition facts (per serving)
Calories 427   Carbohydrate 30g   Protein 35g   Fat 18.1g (of which saturates 5.6g)

Purple Pancetta Penne Serves 4

Preparation time: 10 minutes **Cooking time:** 20 minutes

You can't get a better combination than purple sprouting broccoli and pasta. If you have completed a hard weights session and want some additional dairy protein, you could replace the toasted almonds with feta cheese. This dish can be served hot or cold.

300g/10½oz/3½ cups wholegrain penne pasta
1 tbsp rapeseed/canola oil
1 garlic clove, finely chopped
100g/3½oz pancetta

300g/10½oz purple sprouting broccoli heads
juice of ½ lemon
50g/1¾oz/heaped ¼ cup whole blanched almonds

1 Cook the pasta in a large saucepan of boiling water for 8 minutes, or until tender.

2 Meanwhile, heat the oil in a frying pan over a medium heat, add the garlic and cook for 1 minute, then add the pancetta and fry for about 3 minutes until crisp. Stir in the broccoli heads and lemon juice and cook for a further 3–5 minutes until the broccoli is tender but still crisp.

3 In a small frying pan, toast the almonds for a few minutes until golden.

4 Drain the pasta, then turn it into a serving dish. Add the broccoli and toss together gently. Sprinkle the toasted almonds over the top and serve hot or leave to cool and serve cold.

Nutrition facts (per serving)
Calories 508   Carbohydrate 62g   Protein 26g   Fat 20.3g (of which saturates 3.8g)

Coriander Lamb with Quinoa Serves 4

Preparation time: 15 minutes **Cooking time:** 20 minutes

I'm not a big fan of the term 'super food' but quinoa really is a super grain. Packed full of slow-release carbohydrate and protein, this dish is ideal as a recovery option.

1 tbsp coriander seeds
1 tbsp cumin seeds
1 tbsp olive oil
1 red chilli, deseeded and chopped
juice of ½ orange

400g/14oz canned chickpeas, drained
  and rinsed
100g/3½oz spinach leaves
125g/4½oz/⅔ cup quinoa
4 lamb chops, 50g/2oz each
1 litre/35fl oz/4 cups stock

1 **Preheat the grill/broiler. Put the coriander and cumin seeds in a non-stick frying pan over a medium heat and toast until you can smell their aroma. Transfer to a pestle and mortar and grind to a powder. Blend in the oil, chilli and orange juice to make a paste.**

2 **Brush the spice mix liberally over the chops and grill/broil for 20 minutes, turning and basting regularly, or until the chops are cooked.**

3 **Meanwhile, put the spinach and quinoa in a large saucepan and pour in the stock. Bring to the boil over a high heat, then turn the heat down to low and simmer for 12 minutes until the quinoa is soft. Drain well, then stir in the chickpeas and warm through over a low heat.**

4 **Serve the chops hot on a bed of quinoa.**

Nutrition facts (per serving)
Calories 492   Carbohydrate 57.5g   Protein 35.5g   Fat 13.8g (of which saturates 2.9g)

Lamb & Spinach Curry Serves 4

Preparation time: 15 minutes, plus 30 minutes' marinating **Cooking time:** 1¼ hours

Another spiced-infused, antioxidant-packed curry, this is lovely served with brown rice or wholemeal pitta breads.

2 garlic cloves
4cm/½in piece of root ginger, peeled
   and grated
1 small, very hot green chilli, deseeded
   and thinly sliced
2 handfuls of coriander/cilantro leaves
500g/1lb 2oz boneless shoulder of lamb,
   cut into 2cm/1in pieces

1 tbsp rapeseed/canola oil
1 onion, chopped
1 tsp paprika
½ tsp turmeric
½ tsp salt
4 tbsp fat-free Greek yogurt
400g/14oz baby spinach leaves
4 wholemeal pitta breads, to serve

1 Put the garlic, ginger, chilli and coriander/cilantro into a food processor and blend to a paste. Rub the paste into the lamb, then leave to one side for about 30 minutes to marinate.

2 Heat the oil in a large saucepan over a high heat and cook the onion for about 4 minutes until it is golden and crispy.

3 Add the lamb to the pan, turn the heat down to medium and stir in the paprika, turmeric and salt. Cover and cook for 10 minutes, stirring once or twice. The lamb should shed some water.

4 Add the yogurt 1 tablespoon at a time, stirring each one in before you add the next. Add the spinach and stir for a few minutes until it wilts. Make sure everything is well combined, then cover and turn the heat down as low as possible. Leave to cook for 50 minutes, stirring occasionally, until the lamb is tender.

5 Serve hot with wholemeal pitta breads.

Nutrition facts (per serving)
Calories 495 Carbohydrate 35.2g Protein 42.4g Fat 19.1g (of which saturates 6.4g)

Zesty Mackerel Fillets Serves 4

Preparation time: 15 minutes   **Cooking time:** 25 minutes

Although fish is a common choice for most athletes looking for an easy, lean protein option, oily fish is often overlooked, and yet we should be aiming to consume one or two portions a week to ensure that we meet our omega-3 fat requirements. Mackerel has a strong flavour but combined with all these antioxidant-rich herbs and spices, it works beautifully, providing a well-balanced training meal. You could also serve it with brown rice instead of couscous, if you prefer.

4 mackerel fillets
4cm/1½in piece of root ginger, peeled and
   chopped
2 garlic cloves, finely chopped
1 red chilli, deseeded and finely chopped
300ml/10½fl oz/1¼ cups vegetable stock

200g/7oz/scant 1¼ cups couscous
juice of 1 lime
2 tbsp soy sauce
2 tbsp sweet chilli sauce
1 handful of coriander/cilantro leaves,
   chopped

1 Preheat the oven to 200°C/400°F/Gas 6.

2 Put the mackerel fillets in a single layer in an ovenproof dish. Sprinkle with the ginger, garlic and chilli, then cover with the vegetable stock. Bake for about 20 minutes, or until the fillets flake easily when tested with a fork.

3 After 15 minutes, put the couscous in a bowl and cover with boiling water. Leave to stand, stirring occasionally, until most of the water has been absorbed and the couscous is soft. Drain off any excess water.

4 When the fish is almost cooked, put the lime juice, soy sauce, sweet chilli sauce, ginger and coriander/cilantro in a small saucepan over a low heat.

5 Spoon the couscous onto serving plates and top with the mackerel fillets. Pour the mackerel cooking juices into the saucepan and heat through, then pour the zesty sauce evenly over the mackerel and couscous and serve.

Nutrition facts (per serving)
Calories 443   Carbohydrate 43.5g   Protein 28g   Fat 16.1g (of which saturates 3.3g)

Thai-Style Baked Fish with Stir-Fried Vegetable Rice Serves 4

Preparation time: 15 minutes   **Cooking time:** 20 minutes

Oily fish not only provides vital omega-3 fats but is also a good source of calcium and vitamin D. There have been numerous studies in recent years linking low vitamin D levels with depression, obesity and increased risk of infection in athletes, especially through the winter months. A 100g/3½oz salmon fillet will provide you with 20g of protein and around 80 percent of your daily vitamin D requirements.

4 salmon fillets
zest and juice of 1 lime
1 garlic clove, finely chopped
1 small red chilli, deseeded and chopped
1 tbsp rapeseed/canola oil
1 lemongrass stalk, finely chopped
150g/5½oz baby corn

150g/5½oz mangetout/snow peas or sugar snap peas
150g/5½oz baby carrots
120g/4¼oz/heaped ½ cup brown rice
300ml/10½fl oz/1¼ cups vegetable stock
1 handful of coriander/cilantro leaves, chopped

1 Preheat the oven to 180°C/350°F/Gas 4.

2 Put each fish fillet on a piece of kitchen foil large enough to loosely wrap the fish. Sprinkle with the lime juice, garlic and chilli, then seal the parcels loosely.

3 Bake for 20 minutes, or until the fish flakes easily with a fork.

4 Meanwhile, heat the oil in a wok over a medium heat, add the lemongrass and fry for a minute until you can smell the aroma. Turn the heat up to high, add all the vegetables and stir-fry for 3 minutes.

5 Stir in the rice and pour over the stock. Bring to the boil, then turn the heat down to low and simmer for 15–20 minutes, stirring occasionally, until all the stock has been absorbed and the rice is cooked.

6 Serve the salmon on a bed of rice with the cooking juices spooned over the top. Sprinkle with lime zest and coriander/cilantro to serve.

Nutrition facts (per serving)
Calories 437   Carbohydrate 36g   Protein 39g   Fat 15.8g (of which saturates 2g)

Salmon Pasta Bake <small>Serves 4</small>

Preparation time: 15 minutes   **Cooking time:** 1¼ hours

This is a vitamin D, calcium and omega-3-enriched version of the humble tuna pasta bake that has probably been a staple in your cooking repertoire since you were a student! By adding the extra vegetables and wholemeal pasta, you introduce fibre, making it a complete meal for after training.

300g/10½oz/3 cups dried wholegrain pasta

2 salmon fillets, 120g/4¼oz each

100g/3½oz/¾ cup frozen peas

100g/3½oz/¾ cup frozen sweetcorn/corn kernels

100g/3½oz fresh spinach leaves

2 tbsp plain/all-purpose flour

570ml/20fl oz/2⅓ cups skimmed milk

1 handful of mint leaves, chopped

1 handful of basil leaves, chopped

50g/1¾oz mature/sharp cheese, grated

1 Preheat the oven to 180°C/350°F/Gas 4.

2 Cook the pasta in a large saucepan of boiling water for 8 minutes, or until tender. Drain well, then leave to one side.

3 Meanwhile, put the salmon fillets in an ovenproof dish, cover with kitchen foil and cook in the oven for 10–15 minutes until the salmon flakes easily when tested with a fork. Remove from the oven and lift off the skin. Add the peas, sweetcorn/corn, spinach and cooked pasta to the salmon.

4 Put the flour in a small saucepan and stir in enough of the milk to make a paste. Put the pan over a low heat and whisk in the remaining milk, then stir until the mixture comes to the boil and thickens into a white sauce. Stir in the mint and basil leaves.

5 Pour the sauce over the fish and pasta. Sprinkle the cheese over the top and bake for about 40–45 minutes until the cheese is golden brown and the sauce is bubbling around the edges. Serve straight away.

Nutrition facts (per serving)
Calories 509   Carbohydrate 74.3g   Protein 35g   Fat 10.3g (of which saturates 3.2g)

Easy Fish & Chips Serves 4

Preparation time: 15 minutes   **Cooking time:** 45 minutes

I usually find after a hard race, all I really want is chips/fries. This is my body's way of replacing glycogen stores and electrolytes in the form of salt. By serving the chips/fries with fish, you add protein to help with repair and recovery.

4 fillets of any white or oily fish
zest and juice of 1 lemon
2 large baking potatoes (about 570g/1lb 4oz total weight), sliced into wedges
1 sweet potato, about 300g/10½oz, sliced into wedges
1 tbsp rapeseed/canola oil
½ tsp dried Italian herbs
sea salt and freshly ground black pepper

For the Mushy Peas:
300g/10½oz/heaped 3¼ cups frozen peas
1 tbsp fat-free plain yogurt

For the Lemon Mayonnaise:
2 tbsp fat-free plain yogurt
1 tbsp low-fat mayonnaise
juice of ½ lemon

1 Preheat the oven to 180°C/350°F/Gas 4.

2 Put the fish on a baking sheet and sprinkle with the lemon zest and juice.

3 Put the potato and sweet potato wedges on another baking sheet. Drizzle with the oil, sprinkle with the herbs and season with salt and pepper. Toss to cover them in the seasoned oil. Roast for 20 minutes, or until half cooked.

4 Turn the potatoes with a spatula, then put back in the oven. Put the fish in the oven at the same time and cook both for a further 20 minutes, or until the wedges are crisp and the fish flakes easily when tested with a fork.

5 Meanwhile, cook the peas in boiling water for about 3 minutes, then drain well. Blend the peas with the yogurt and 1 tablespoon water to produce a soft, mushy-pea texture.

6 Mix together the yogurt, mayonnaise and lemon juice to make the Lemon Mayonnaise.

7 Serve the fish, wedges and peas with the Lemon Mayonnaise.

Nutrition facts (per serving)
Calories 471   Carbohydrate 61g   Protein 22g   Fat 16.8g (of which saturates 3.8g)

Magic Fish Pie Serves 4

Preparation time: 20 minutes   **Cooking time:** 1 hour

My children love this version of fish pie. In fact they don't seem to enjoy fish any other way! Once again, to save time, I have added vegetables to the main dish and also sneaked a few into the topping. This helps to reduce the carbohydrate content of the meal. The skimmed-milk sauce, the mixed fish and the cheese topping make the pie an ideal choice after a hard strength and conditioning or weights session or a moderate workout.

1 sweet potato (about 300g/10½oz), chopped
2 large carrots, sliced
1 large parsnip, peeled and chopped
670ml/23fl oz/2⅔ cups skimmed milk
60g/2oz low-fat cream cheese with chives
2 tbsp plain/all-purpose flour
1 smoked haddock fillet, cut into bite-size chunks

1 smoked mackerel fillet, cut into bite-size chunks
1 salmon fillet, cut into bite-size chunks
300g/10½oz mixed vegetables, such as frozen peas, sweetcorn/corn kernels and spinach

1 Preheat the oven to 180°C/350°F/Gas 4.

2 Put the sweet potato, carrots and parsnip in a large saucepan, cover with water and bring to the boil over a high heat. Turn the heat down to low and simmer for 10 minutes, or until tender. Drain, then mash with 100ml/3½fl oz/generous ⅓ cup of the milk and the cream cheese.

3 Put the flour in a small saucepan and stir in enough of the milk to make a paste. Put the pan over a low heat and whisk in the remaining milk, then stir until the mixture comes to the boil and thickens into a white sauce.

4 Put the fish pieces into the bottom of a large ovenproof dish and add the mixed vegetables. Pour the sauce over the top and stir together gently. Spread the mash mixture over the top.

5 Bake for 30–40 minutes until the pie is piping hot and the top is crisp. Serve straight away.

Nutrition facts (per serving)
Calories 353   Carbohydrate 32g   Protein 20g   Fat 13.6g (of which saturates 5g)

Rosemary & Paprika Vegetable & Bean Hot Pot Serves 4

Preparation time: 15 minutes **Cooking time:** 1 hour

I have to admit this is one of my favourite recipes. It is full of goodness from the vegetables, and the pulses add a good source of protein for vegetarians as well as iron, calcium and B vitamins. If you are planning on a moderate or hard training session the following day, or have just completed one, then serve the hot pot with toast or even a baked potato, but if it is a rest day, this is just as satisfying served alone as a chunky soup.

2 garlic cloves, finely chopped
4cm/1½in piece of root ginger, peeled and chopped
2 large courgettes/zucchini, cut into chunks
2 large carrots, cut into chunks
200g/7oz broccoli florets
200g/7oz green beans, halved
400g/14oz canned chopped tomatoes
400g/14oz canned chickpeas, drained and rinsed

400g/14oz canned red kidney beans, drained and rinsed
1 tsp salt
2 tsp paprika
1 tsp soft light brown sugar
2 handfuls of rosemary leaves
sea salt and freshly ground black pepper
sourdough toast or baked potato, to serve (optional)

1 Preheat the oven to 180°C/350°F/Gas 4.

2 Put all the ingredients in a large casserole dish and pour in 400ml/14fl oz/generous 1½ cups water. Cover and bake for 1 hour, or until all the vegetables are cooked through and some of the juice has been absorbed.

3 Ladle into dishes and serve with slices of sourdough toast or a baked potato, if you like.

Nutrition facts (per serving without toast or potato)
Calories 515   Carbohydrate 94g   Protein 30g   Fat 5g (of which saturates 0.4g)

Sweet Potato Risotto Serves 4

Preparation time: 10 minutes **Cooking time:** 20 minutes

An ideal choice before a long endurance day or race day, the protein in a traditional risotto has been removed and replaced with extra slow-release carbohydrate in the form of sweet potato to ensure that your glycogen stores are full. This dish also travels well, so if you are doing an event away from home and are able to reheat food, this is a good option to take with you.

300g/10½oz/1¾ cups basmati rice
2 sweet potatoes (about 600g/1lb 5oz total weight), peeled and chopped
750ml/26fl oz/3 cups vegetable stock
1 tbsp rapeseed/canola oil
1 garlic clove, finely chopped
2.5cm/1in piece of root ginger, peeled and finely chopped

250g/9oz stir-fry vegetables of your choice, such as baby corn, courgettes/zucchini and mangetout/snow peas/sugar snap peas
juice of 1 lime
1 tbsp sweet chilli sauce
1 tbsp soy sauce
1 handful of coriander/cilantro leaves, chopped

1 Put the rice and sweet potatoes in a large saucepan, pour over the stock and bring to the boil over a high heat. Turn the heat down to low and simmer for about 10 minutes until all the stock has been absorbed and both the rice and sweet potatoes are tender. Add a little more boiling water if necessary.

2 Heat the oil in a wok over a high heat. Add the garlic, ginger and vegetables and stir-fry for 3–5 minutes until the vegetables are tender but still crisp. Add the lime juice, chilli sauce and soy sauce. Stir in the rice and sweet potato mixture and stir-fry for a further 3 minutes until everything is hot and well mixed.

3 Serve hot, sprinkled with coriander/cilantro.

Nutrition facts (per serving)
Calories 423   Carbohydrate 87g   Protein 7g   Fat 4.1g (of which saturates 0.4g)

Tofu Pad Thai Serves 4

Preparation time: 15 minutes   **Cooking time:** 15 minutes

This is one of my all-time favourite dishes – I have combined all the aspects of a Thai menu that I like best and come up with this gem of a dish. I have served this to many of my running friends and it has always gone down a treat! It makes a great pre- or post- endurance training meal.

1 tbsp vegetable oil
1 garlic clove, finely chopped
1cm/½in piece of root ginger, peeled and finely chopped
2 tbsp red curry paste
400g/14oz mixed stir-fry veg of choice such as baby corn, sugar snap peas, carrots

2 packets pre-cooked straight-to-wok egg noodles
200g/7oz smoked tofu
400g/14oz can chickpeas, drained and rinsed
400ml/14oz can coconut milk
1 large handful coriander/cilantro leaves, chopped

1 Heat the oil in a large wok and add the garlic and ginger. Cook until golden brown, then add the red curry paste. Cook for a further 3 minutes until the aroma of the spices is released.

2 Add the vegetables and stir-fry for 5 minutes, then add the noodles and continue to stir-fry for another 3 minutes.

3 Add the tofu and chickpeas and pour over the coconut milk. Cook for a further 2 minutes to warm the chickpeas and milk through. Stir in the coriander/cilantro and serve immediately.

Nutrition facts (per serving)
Calories 530   Carbohydrate 45g   Protein 16.6g;   Fat 30.1g (of which saturates 17g)

Punjabi-Style Aloo Sabsi Serves 4

Preparation time: 15 minutes   **Cooking time:** 25 minutes

Aloo sabsi is translated from the Punjabi as 'potato curry'. I grew up on this dish as a fussy child who did not like her vegetables! However, in recent years I have chosen to include this as a great option before an endurance event as it's a novel way of including more carbohydrate, especially if served with rice or chappatis. This dish can also be eaten cold, making it great as a portable snack on long bike rides, wrapped in a chappati or even in a wholemeal pitta bread.

1 tbsp rapeseed/canola oil

2 tsp cumin seeds

2 tsp black mustard seeds

1kg/2lb 4oz floury potatoes, such as Maris Piper, cut into chunks

400g/14oz canned chopped tomatoes

¾ tsp salt

1 tsp garam masala

¼–½ tsp chilli powder

½ tsp turmeric

juice of ½ lemon

1 Heat the oil in a large wok or balti dish over a high heat. Add the cumin and mustard seeds and stir-fry for 1 minute until you can smell their aroma. Add the potatoes and stir-fry for 3–5 minutes until coated with seeds.

2 Add the tomatoes, salt, garam masala, chilli powder, turmeric and lemon juice and mix together so the potatoes are covered in sauce and spices. Stir in 400ml/14fl oz/ generous 1½ cups water. Cover and bring to the boil, then turn the heat down to low and simmer for 10–15 minutes until the potatoes are cooked and there is little juice left. Serve hot or cold.

Nutrition facts (per serving)
Calories 221   Carbohydrate 44g   Protein 5.1g   Fat 3.9g (of which saturates 0.8g)

Bulgar Wheat Curry Serves 4

Preparation time: 15 minutes   **Cooking time:** 1 hour

This is an excellent vegan recovery meal, although you don't need to be vegan to enjoy it. The combination of grain and pulses creates a whole protein with all the essential amino acids usually found in animal protein.

1 tbsp rapeseed/canola oil
2 garlic cloves, finely chopped
1 onion, chopped
2 celery stalks, chopped
1 tsp ground cumin
1 tsp chilli powder
1 red pepper, deseeded and chopped
1 carrot, chopped
1 courgette/zucchini, chopped

400g/14oz canned kidney beans, drained
   and rinsed
400g/14oz canned aduki beans, drained
   and rinsed
125g/4½oz/⅔ cup bulgar wheat
1 handful of coriander/cilantro leaves,
   chopped
sea salt and freshly ground black pepper

1 Heat the oil in a large pan over a medium heat. Add the garlic and onion and fry for 3 minutes, or until golden brown. Add the celery, cumin and chilli powder and cook for a further 5 minutes, stirring regularly.

2 Add the pepper, carrot and courgette/zucchini and cook for 10 minutes, or until all the vegetables are tender. Add a little water if they start to stick to the pan.

3 Add both types of beans, the bulgar wheat and 500ml/17fl oz/2 cups water. Bring to the boil over a high heat, then turn the heat down to low and simmer for 30–40 minutes until the water has been absorbed.

4 Season to taste with salt and pepper and serve sprinkled with the coriander/cilantro.

Nutrition facts (per serving)
Calories 361   Carbohydrate 61g   Protein 19g   Fat 4.3g (of which saturates 0.8g)

Sweet Potato Parcels Serves 4

Preparation time: 5 minutes   **Cooking time:** 1 hour

The slow-release energy from sweet potatoes has been well documented for many years. This recipe is ideal for either before or after training. Feta is a lower-fat dairy option, which provides protein and calcium. Diets of individuals with high-calcium intakes from low-fat dairy sources have been linked with accretion of more lean muscle mass than in individuals with lower intake, making this dish a winning choice.

4 sweet potatoes (about 1.2kg/2lb 12oz total weight)

1 bunch of spring onions/scallions, chopped

100g/3½oz feta cheese, crumbled

green salad leaves, cherry tomatoes and toasted seeds, to serve

1 Preheat the oven to 200°C/400°F/Gas 6. Pierce each sweet potato several times with a fork, then bake for 40–45 minutes until cooked through and tender. Remove from the oven and cut in half.

2 Preheat the grill/broiler to medium. Very carefully, use a spoon to scoop out the sweet potato flesh, keeping the skins intact. Mix the flesh with the spring onions/scallions and feta cheese, then spoon the mixture back into the empty skins.

3 Grill/broil the sweet potatoes for 5–10 minutes until golden brown. Serve with a tomato and toasted seed salad.

Nutrition facts (per serving)

Calories 421   Carbohydrate 85g   Protein 8g   Fat 5.8g (of which saturates 3.9g)

HERO FOOD: SWEET POTATO

Sweet potatoes have taken over in popularity from the humble white potato due to their high beta-carotene content and because they are a great source of complex carbohydrate, providing slow release energy and making it an ideal fuel before or after exercise. They are perfect baked and served with oily fish as a recovery meal or added to a risotto for a pre-endurance training meal. Add them to salads or make soup for great lunch options, helping to prevent that 4pm sugar slump. They are a must in every athlete's storecupboard.

Mixed Nut Pesto & Roasted Mediterranean Vegetable Pasta Serves 4

Preparation time: 15 minutes   **Cooking time:** 45 minutes

I couldn't leave the pasta lovers out! This dish is suitable for vegans as the pesto is made without cheese. I have used coriander/cilantro leaves, but you could opt for the more traditional basil, if you prefer.

250g/9oz wholegrain pasta
½ tbsp rapeseed/canola oil
sea salt and freshly ground black pepper

For the Mixed Nut Pesto:
100g/3½oz/⅔ cup mixed unsalted nuts
1 tbsp tahini
100g/3½oz coriander/cilantro leaves
juice of 1 lemon
2 garlic cloves

For the Roasted Mediterranean Vegetables:
2 aubergines/eggplants, sliced
2 courgettes/zucchini, sliced
1 red pepper, deseeded and cut into chunks
1 yellow pepper, deseeded and cut into chunks
2 garlic cloves
300g/10½oz mushrooms
1 tbsp rapeseed/canola oil
1 tsp dried oregano
1 tsp dried Italian herbs

1 Preheat the oven to 180°C/350°F/Gas 4.

2 To make the pesto, put all the ingredients into a blender or food processor and pulse gently until the nuts have been broken down but the overall consistency of the pesto is still quite rough rather than a smooth paste.

3 Put all the vegetables onto a baking sheet. Sprinkle with the oil and herbs and toss together gently. Bake for 30–40 minutes until the vegetables are crisp and browned.

4 Meanwhile, cook the pasta in a large saucepan of boiling water for 10 minutes, or until tender. Drain well, then toss with the oil to prevent it from sticking together. Leave to one side.

5 Mix the pesto into the cooked pasta and serve hot.

Nutrition facts (per serving)
Calories 538   Carbohydrate 73g   Protein 21g   Fat 21g (of which saturates 2.6g)

SNACKS & PORTABLES

Dark Chocolate & Ginger Muffins

Makes 12 muffins

Preparation time: 15 minutes   **Cooking time:** 15 minutes

I do not generally advocate cakes, biscuits/cookies, desserts and sweet things. However, I have always believed that these foods can be included in moderation in a healthy balanced diet. Muffins are easy to make and I have reduced the fat and sugar content of these without affecting the flavour. Serve them with a milk-based drink as a recovery option or take them on bike rides, trail runs or hikes to keep energy levels topped up.

200g/7oz/1²⁄₃ cups self-raising/
   self-rising flour
½ tsp baking powder
2 eggs, beaten
3 tbsp rapeseed/canola oil
100ml/3½fl oz/generous ⅓ cup
   skimmed milk

1 tsp vanilla extract
50g/1¾oz/heaped ¼ cup light soft
   brown sugar
75g/2½oz dark/bittersweet chocolate with
   ginger pieces, broken into chunks
2cm/¾in piece of root ginger, peeled
   and grated

1 Preheat the oven to 180°C/350°F/Gas 4 and line a 12-hole muffin pan with paper cases.

2 Sift the flour and baking powder together into a large bowl. Beat the eggs, oil, milk, vanilla and sugar together in a separate bowl.

3 Gently fold the liquid mixture into the flour mixture but do not over-mix. Add the chocolate chunks and grated ginger and fold together gently until just combined.

4 Spoon the mixture into the prepared cases and bake for 15 minutes until the muffins are well risen and the tops spring back when lightly pressed with the fingertips.

5 Transfer to a wire rack to cool. Store in an airtight container for up to 3 days.

Nutrition facts (per muffin)
Calories 155   Carbohydrate 20g   Protein 3.3g   Fat 6.7g (of which saturates 2.1g)

Carrot & Ginger Cake Makes 18 slices

Preparation time: 15 minutes   Cooking time: 1 hour

Carrot cake is one of my favourites, so I modified the recipe so that it can also work as a great pre-training option. The wholemeal flour ensures that it is a good source of slow-release carbohydrate, while the blend of ginger and mixed spice give this cake real depth.

150ml/5fl oz/⅔ cup walnut oil, plus extra for greasing
6 eggs
150g/5½oz/heaped ¾ cup dark soft brown sugar
2 tsp mixed/apple pie spice
½ tsp vanilla extract

450g/1lb/3⅔ cups wholemeal self-raising/self-rising flour
500g/1lb 2oz carrots, grated
200g/7oz/1⅓ cups raisins
150g/5½oz/scant 1¼ cups walnuts
1cm/½in piece of root ginger, peeled and grated

1 Preheat the oven to 180°C/350°F/Gas 4 and grease a 20cm/8in cake pan.

2 Beat together the oil, eggs, sugar, spice and vanilla until well mixed. Fold in the remaining ingredients until just mixed.

3 Pour into the prepared cake pan and bake for 1 hour, or until a knife inserted in the centre comes out clean.

4 Transfer to a wire rack to cool. Store in an airtight container for up to 3 days.

Nutrition facts (per slice)
Calories 257   Carbohydrate 36.5g   Protein 8.3g   Fat 9.5g (of which saturates 0.9g)

Courgette Tea Bread Makes 12 slices

Preparation time: 15 minutes **Cooking time:** 30 minutes

This tea bread has a slight twist on the traditional recipe. I like to use fruit and vegetables in cakes whenever possible and this is no exception. This time I have used courgette/zucchini.

3 tbsp rapeseed/canola oil, plus extra for greasing
85g/3oz/scant ⅓ cup clear honey
2 eggs
150ml/5fl oz/⅔ cup cooled chai tea
zest of 1 lemon
250g/9oz/1⅔ cups wholemeal spelt flour

1 tsp bicarbonate of soda/baking soda
¼ tsp baking powder
a pinch of salt
250g/9oz courgette/zucchini, grated
50g/1¾oz/ chopped mixed nuts
50g/1¾oz/heaped ⅓ cup raisins
a little butter, to serve

1 Preheat the oven to 180°C/350°F/Gas 4 and grease a 450g/1lb loaf pan.

2 Whisk together the oil, honey, eggs, tea and lemon zest until light and fluffy. Sift in the flour, bicarbonate of soda/baking soda, baking powder and salt, then gently fold it into the honey mixture. Swirl in the courgettes/zucchini, nuts and raisins but don't over-mix.

3 Pour into the prepared loaf pan and bake for 25–30 minutes until a knife inserted in the centre comes out clean.

4 Transfer the tea bread to a wire rack to cool. Slice and serve on its own or spread with a thin layer of butter.

Nutrition facts (per slice without butter)
Calories 127 Carbohydrate 16g Protein 3g Fat 6.9g (of which saturates 1.1g)

Sweet Potato Brownies Makes 15 brownies

Preparation time: 15 minutes   **Cooking time:** 25 minutes

When I tell my athletes I have a recipe for brownies they are allowed to eat, their faces light up. This healthy version is low in fat and packed with slow-release carbohydrates in the form of sweet potatoes – a great snack to be eaten 1–2 hours before a training session or competition. Enjoyed with a glass of milk, they are also a good way to start replacing glycogen stores after a training session. Try replacing the cherries with dark chocolate chunks and walnuts for broken up brazil nuts, or experiment with your favourite dried fruit and nuts.

1 small sweet potato (about 225g/8oz)
100g/3½oz low-fat margarine
100g/3½oz dark/bittersweet chocolate, (at least 70% cocoa solids), broken into chunks
100g/3½oz/½ cup dark soft brown sugar
2 eggs

1 tsp vanilla extract
100g/3½oz/heaped ¾ cup plain/all-purpose flour
¼ tsp baking powder
50g/1¾oz/heaped ⅓ cup sour cherries
75g/2½oz/heaped ½ cup walnuts, roughly chopped

1 Preheat the oven to 200°C/400°F/Gas 6.

2 Pierce the potato with a fork and bake for 1 hour, or until soft. Leave until cool enough to handle, then scoop out the flesh into a bowl. You should have about 200g/7oz. While it is cooling, turn the oven down to 180°C/350°F/Gas 4 and line an 18cm/7in square cake pan with baking paper or kitchen foil.

3 Melt the margarine in a saucepan over a low heat, add the chocolate and stir until half melted, then remove from the heat and stir until melted.

4 Add the sugar to the sweet potato and beat until almost smooth. Stir in the margarine and chocolate, eggs and vanilla and beat until thick. Fold in the flour and baking powder, then the cherries and walnuts.

5 Spoon into the prepared pan, smooth the top and bake for 20–25 minutes until a crust forms on the top but the brownie is still soft under the crust. Leave to cool completely in the pan before slicing.

Nutrition facts (per brownie)
Calories 172   Carbohydrate 20g   Protein 3.5g   Fat 8.9g (of which saturates 2.7g)

Coconut Energy Bites Makes 30 bites

Preparation time: 15 minutes

This recipe was devised by a good friend of mine, Nick or, as he is sometimes known, Mr Seven Hills Chocolate! After we discussed the idea of an energy bar while away on a trail running week, Nick developed this and and has allowed me to use the recipe here. Each bite is full of energy and ideal for long bikes or runs as an alternative to gels or jelly babies. They also go well with coffee, so are ideal for recovery if combined with a latte.

100g/3½oz/1 cup blanched almonds
100g/3½oz/1 cup pecan nuts
250g/9oz/1½ cups Medjool dates, pitted
200g/7oz/2½ cups desiccated/dried shredded coconut
30g/1oz/2 tbsp chia seeds
50g/1¾oz/⅓ cup raisins
30g/1oz/¼ cup cocoa powder

40g/1½oz/⅓ cup cocoa nibs
a pinch of salt
a pinch of ground cinnamon
90g/3¼oz/⅓ cup coconut oil
100g/3½oz good-quality dark/bittersweet chocolate (at least 70% cocoa solids), broken into chunks

1 Line a 30 x 25cm/12 x 10in baking pan with baking parchment.

2 Put the nuts in a frying pan and dry toast for a few minutes over a medium heat until golden. Blitz the toasted nuts in a food processor for a couple of minutes until you have a chunky paste. Add all the remaining ingredients except the coconut oil and dark chocolate to the food processor and blitz for 1–2 minutes until it all comes together.

3 Put the chocolate and coconut oil in a heatproof bowl and rest it over a pan of gently simmering water, making sure the bottom of the bowl does not touch the water. Heat, stirring occasionally, until the chocolate and oil have melted. Add the melted mixture to the food processor and blitz to blend everything together.

4 Tip the mixture into the prepared pan and put in the refrigerator for 3 hours until chilled and firm. Scoop out spoonfuls about the size a **large walnut** and mould with your hands into balls and you are good to go! Store in an airtight container in the fridge for up to 5 days.

Nutrition facts (per bite)
Calories 173   Carbohydrate 14g   Protein 2.4g   Fat 1.3g (of which saturates 1.5g)

Choco-Nut Banana Bread Makes 8 slices

Preparation time: 20 minutes **Cooking time:** 40 minutes

This lovely banana bread makes a great companion with a glass of milk or latte post run as a recovery option; or mid afternoon as a carbohydrate top up prior to an evening run session.

butter or oil, for greasing
100g/3½oz/1 cup oats
50g/1¾oz/2½ tbsp honey
75g/2½oz/5 tbsp smooth peanut butter
2 eggs

50g/1¾oz/⅓ cup dark chocolate chunks
3 ripe bananas, mashed
100g/3½oz/¾ cup spelt flour
2½ tsp baking powder

1 Preheat the oven to 180°C/350°F/Gas 4 and grease a 500g/1lb loaf pan.

2 Put the oats in a food processor and blend until finely ground.

3 In a large mixing bowl, mix together the honey and peanut butter.

4 Beat in the eggs, then stir in the chocolate chunks, mashed banana and 4 tablespoons water.

5 Sift in the ground oats, flour and baking powder, and fold the ingredients together until all mixed in.

6 Pour the batter into the prepared loaf pan and bake in the preheated oven for 30–40 minutes until cooked all the way through. Allow to cool for a few minutes in the pan, then turn out onto a wire rack to cool completely. Cut into 8 slices to serve.

Nutrition facts (per square)
Calories 254 Carbohydrate 39.2 Protein 8.1g Fat 8.9g (of which saturates 1.2g)

Banana & Nut Butter Sandwich Serves 1

Preparation time: 5 minutes

Some flavours just go together naturally. Banana and nuts is one such combination, so I have brought them together here in this nourishing snack – perfect to accompany your recovery milkshake or smoothie.

1 banana
2 tsp Nut Butter (see page 131) made with
   almonds, or nut butter of your choice

1 Slice the banana in half lengthways.

2 Spread the Nut Butter across one half of banana and then replace the top like a sandwich. This snack can be eaten straight away or wrapped and transported for later.

Nutrition facts (per serving)
Calories 169   Carbohydrate 29g   Protein 3.4g   Fat 6g (of which saturates 0.6g)

HERO FOOD: NUT BUTTER

Most athletes are surprised when I mention they can eat nut butters. Yes they are high in fat, but they are high in good fats and provide you with so many other essential nutrients, too, such as calcium, iron, magnesium, phosphorus and vitamin E. The high fat content means they help to keep you full and so can actually be useful for people who are trying to lose or watch their weight – but do be careful about quantity! Nuts also provide protein, so they can be particularly useful in vegan and vegetarian diets. One thing to watch, though – they don't make such a good choice post a high-intensity training session as the fat content means that it slows down the absorption of protein needed for recovery. One way round this is to have a glass of milk first (soya if you are vegan), and follow up with your nut butter!

Pepper & Yogurt Dip Serves 6

Preparation time: 5 minutes, plus chilling **Cooking time:** 15 minutes

This is originally my mum, Katy's recipe. My mum has been a huge inspiration to me in many ways and has definitely influenced my culinary skills. She is an amazing cook and has taught me the importance of patience and using spice skilfully! This recipe is fantastic as a high-protein vegetarian dip alternative to hummus. Additionally it is a good way to use up yogurt that has gone slightly sour.

2 tsp rapeseed/canola oil
1 tsp black mustard seeds
1 green pepper, deseeded and chopped

1 red pepper, deseeded and chopped
30g/1oz/heaped ¼ cup gram (chickpea) flour
500g/1lb 2oz/2 cups fat-free plain yogurt

1 Heat the oil in a non-stick frying pan over a medium heat. Add the mustard seeds and fry for 1 minute, or until they start popping. Add the peppers and cook for 5 minutes, or until soft.

2 Stir in the gram flour and cook for 2 minutes, stirring continuously, until the flour has blended into the peppers. Turn the heat up to medium, add the yogurt and bring to the boil, then turn the heat down to low and simmer for about 5 minutes until the yogurt has a thick and paste-like consistency.

3 Transfer to a bowl and leave to cool, then cover with cling film/plastic wrap and chill in the fridge. Store for up to 5 days.

Nutrition facts (per serving)
Calories 113 Carbohydrate 10g Protein 5g Fat 5.5g (of which saturates 1.2g)

Mackerel Pâté Serves 4

Preparation time: 5 minutes

Mackerel is an oily fish and therefore an excellent source of omega-3 fats, calcium and vitamin D. The cream cheese and yogurt soften its strong flavour and make this a nutritious topping for oatcakes, or even a great wrap filling.

2 peppered smoked mackerel fillets,
   skinned
2 tbsp low-fat cream cheese

2 tbsp fat-free Greek yogurt
juice of 1 lemon
oatcakes, to serve

1 Put all the ingredients in a food processor and pulse until smooth.

2 Spoon into a bowl, cover with cling film/plastic wrap and chill in the fridge before serving. It will keep for up to 2 days.

Nutrition facts (per serving)
Calories 181 Carbohydrate 1.6g Protein 10g Fat 14.7g (of which saturates 4.5g)

Spinach & Parmesan Muffins

Makes 12 muffins

Preparation time: 15 minutes   **Cooking time:** 15 minutes

These muffins are great as an alternative to a sandwich for lunch, as an accompaniment to soup for a light meal or even to keep up your energy on a long bike ride, trail run or hike instead of the usual sweet options on offer.

a little rapeseed/canola oil, for greasing
125g/4½oz spinach leaves, chopped
150g/5½oz/scant 1¼ cups plain/all purpose wholemeal flour
1 tsp baking powder
a pinch of sea salt and freshly ground black pepper

2 eggs
80ml/2½fl oz/⅓ cup skimmed milk
3 tbsp white wine vinegar
2 tbsp olive oil
100g/3½oz Parmesan or mature/sharp Cheddar cheese, finely grated

1 Preheat the oven to 220°C/425°F/Gas 7 and grease a 12-hole muffin pan.

2 Put the spinach in a steamer over a saucepan of boiling water, cover and steam for 2 minutes until wilted. Drain and leave to one side.

3 Mix together the flour, baking powder and salt in a large bowl and season with pepper. Add the eggs, milk, vinegar and oil and stir until just combined. Fold in the spinach and grated cheese but do not over-mix.

4 Spoon the mixture into the prepared muffin pan and bake for 15 minutes, or well risen and slightly springy to the touch.

5 Transfer to a wire rack to cool slightly, then serve warm or cold. Store in an airtight container for up to 3 days.

Nutrition facts (per muffin)
Carbohydrate 7.8g   Protein 5.6g   Fat 5.1g (of which saturates 1.8g)

Cheese & Chilli Scones Makes 12 Scones

Preparation time: 20 minutes   **Cooking time:** 12 minutes

These lightly spiced scones are great served with soup or even a casserole or stew. They are good for lunch boxes and make a nutritious alternative to sweet bars and cakes on long endurance-training sessions.

low-calorie cooking oil spray, for greasing
350g/12oz/2¾ cups self-raising/self-rising wholemeal flour, plusextra for dusting
1 tsp baking powder
½ tsp salt
3 tbsp rapeseed/canola oil

50g/1¾oz mature/sharp Cheddar cheese, grated
1 tsp dried chilli/hot pepper flakes
100g/3½oz/scant ½ cup fat-free Greek yogurt
100ml/3½fl oz/scant ½ cup skimmed milk

1 Preheat the oven to 220°C/425°F/Gas 7 and lightly grease a large baking sheet.

2 Put the flour, baking powder, salt and oil in a bowl and bring together until the mixture resembles breadcrumbs. Stir in the cheese and chilli/hot pepper flakes and make a well in the centre. Add the yogurt and half the milk and bring the mixture together to produce a soft dough.

3 Turn the dough out onto a lightly floured surface and shape into a ball, then roll out to about 2cm/¾in thick. Cut into 12 rounds using a 6cm/2½in biscuit/cookie cutter, lightly re-rolling the trimmings until all the dough has been used.

4 Put the scones on the prepared baking sheet and brush the tops with the remaining milk. Bake for 10–12 minutes until risen and golden in colour.

5 Transfer to a wire rack to cool. Store in an airtight container for up to 3 days.

Nutrition facts (per scone)
Calories 136   Carbohydrate 17g   Protein 5g   Fat 5.4g (of which saturates 1.6g)

Easy Snack Suggestions

Sometimes it is not possible to make all your own portable snacks or recovery options, so here are a few ideas for products that you can buy or make very quickly to help with your overall training nutrition.

Flavoured milk – any flavour
Milk-based drinks, such as lattes
Cereal bars – there are many on the market but some are better than others. The ones I tend to recommend to my athletes are:
    Chia Charge bars (from www.running food.co.uk)
    9 bars – all varieties (from most supermarkets and health-food stores)
    Nakd bars – all varieties (from most supermarkets and health-food stores)
    Trek bars – all varieties (from most supermarkets and health-food stores)
Clif bars and shots
Dried fruit and nut mixes
Salted peanuts
Sachets of peanut butter, such as Pip & Nut or Whole Earth
Jelly Babies or jelly cubes
Gels – good options include TORQ, Clif or SiS, but most important is using ones you can tolerate.
Slices of malt loaf
Seeded or sweetened oatcakes

RECOVERY DRINKS

Often after a hard training session, appetites can actually be suppressed at first, but it is also the most important time to take in nutrients to help with the recovery process. Having a drink could be the best solution as not only will it start replacing carbohydrate and protein, it will also help with rehydration. The general rule of thumb for a recovery drink is that it should be 3:1 carbohydrate to protein. The easiest way to achieve this is to use a milk-based option. A lot of the protein shakes and recovery drinks on the market are actually just glorified milk. Why not save some money and make your own tastier versions such as those included in this section? To make the perfect latte all you need is 1 shot of strong espresso topped with 250ml/9fl oz/1 cup warm milk.

Tropical Smoothie Serves 1

Preparation time: 5 minutes

This is so easy to make, but I usually suggest to my athletes that they have it ready in the fridge so they can drink it as soon as they get back from training – or you can have the ingredients waiting in a blender ready to turn on as soon as you step through the door! The Greek yogurt ensures that recovery protein requirements are met.

200ml/7fl oz/¾ cup tropical fruit juice
200g/7oz/¾ cup fat-free Greek yogurt
1 handful of ice

Put all ingredients in a blender and blend until smooth. Pour into a glass and serve straight away.

Nutrition facts (per serving)
Calories 239 Carbohydrate 38g Protein 20g Fat 0g (of which saturates 0g)

Mocha Shake Serves 1

Preparation time: 5 minutes

One of my favourite recovery drinks, especially after a tough session on a hot day. Coconut water is known for its rehydration properties.

3 tsp unsweetened cocoa powder
1 tsp sugar
1 tsp instant coffee powder

300ml/10½fl oz/1¼ cups skimmed milk
200ml/7fl oz/¾ cup coconut water
1 handful of ice

Put all ingredients into a blender and blend until smooth. Pour into a glass and serve straight away.

Nutrition facts (per serving)
Calories 140   Carbohydrate 25g   Protein 10g   Fat 0g (of which saturates 0g)

Recovery Hot Chocolate Serves 1

Preparation time: 5 minutes   **Cooking time:** 5 minutes

This indulgent drink contains the right balance of carbohydrate and protein for recovery. It's amazing after a cold, late training session.

300ml/10½fl oz/1¼ cups skimmed milk
25g/1oz skimmed milk powder

20g/¾oz dark/bittersweet chocolate (at least 70% cocoa solids), broken into chunks

1 **Put the milk and milk powder in a saucepan over a low heat, stirring occasionally, until the powder has dissolved into the milk. Add the chocolate and keep stirring until the chocolate has melted.**

2 **Pour into a mug and serve straight away.**

Nutrition facts (per serving)
Calories 290   Carbohydrate 39g   Protein 19g   Fat 6.1g (of which saturates 4.3g)

DESSERTS

Frozen Vanilla Yogurt Serves 4

Preparation time: 10 minutes, plus at least 4 hours' freezing

Most of us feel the need for a sweet treat after a main meal. This recipe helps you meet your calcium requirements and daily protein intake – as well as being delicious.

600g/1lb 5oz fat-free Greek yogurt
1 tsp vanilla extract
2 tbsp clear honey

1 vanilla pod/bean, split lengthways and
seeds scraped out

1 Put the yogurt, vanilla extract and honey in a large bowl and stir in the vanilla seeds. Spoon the mixture into a 450g/1lb loaf pan, cover with cling film/plastic wrap and put in the freezer for at least 4 hours. Alternatively, you can freeze the yogurt in individual pots.

2 Take out of the freezer 10–15 minutes before serving to allow the dessert to soften.

Nutrition facts (per serving)
Calories 121   Carbohydrate 15g   Protein 16g   Fat 0g (of which saturates 0g)

HERO FOOD: GREEK YOGURT

I'm a great fan of yogurt as a recovery option, but I particularly favour fat-free Greek yogurt because of its high protein content. Most plain Greek yogurt provides 10g of protein per 100g/3½oz yogurt, which is double the amount found in standard yogurts. Protein is an important nutrient required in the recovery process in order to repair and rebuild muscles, helping them to adapt to the training process. Greek yogurt is an ideal choice due to its versatility – it can be mixed into fruit, added to smoothies, or eaten with cereal such as muesli or granola. You can also use it as a base for a slightly more decadent dessert, meaning you can enjoy your pudding guilt free, knowing that it is also the perfect recovery food.

Berry & Toasted Almond Pots Serves 4

Preparation time: 10 minutes, plus cooling **Cooking time:** 10 minutes

I like having friends over for dinner but I still see this an as opportunity to fuel my training correctly, which is why I came up with this recipe. It delivers on taste, looks beautiful and also continues to work as training food for me!

50g/1¾oz/heaped ⅓ cup flaked/slivered almonds

500g/1lb 2oz mixed berries, fresh or frozen, defrosted

400g/14oz fat-free Greek yogurt

4 heaped tsp clear honey

1 Put the flaked/slivered almonds in a dry frying pan over a medium heat and toss for a few minutes until just beginning to brown. Tip out and leave to one side.

2 Put the berries in a saucepan with 4 tablespoons water over a medium heat, bring to the boil, then turn the heat down to low and simmer for 10 minutes, or until the berries are soft and cooked with some juice remaining. Leave to cool slightly.

3 Spoon the berries into tall glasses or ice-cream bowls. Spoon the yogurt over the top, then drizzle 1 teaspoon honey over the top of each portion. Top each bowl with some toasted flaked/slivered almonds and serve. This dessert can also be kept in the fridge until ready to serve.

Nutrition facts (per serving)
Calories 241   Carbohydrate 27g   Protein 15g   Fat 8.7g (of which saturates 0.6g)

Nectarine Compôte with Zesty Crème Fraîche Serves 4

Preparation time: 10 minutes, plus 10 minutes' cooling   **Cooking time:** 15 minutes

The combination of flavours in this fruit-based dessert make it a decadent and yet guilt-free post-dinner sweet treat.

4 large, ripe nectarines, quartered and
   pitted
zest and juice of 1 orange

1 tbsp dark soft brown sugar
1 tsp grated root ginger
120g/4¼oz/½ cup low-fat crème fraîche

1 Put the nectarines, orange juice, sugar and ginger in a saucepan with 3 tablespoons water over a low heat and cook gently for 10 minutes, or until the nectarines are soft.

2 Lift out the nectarine quarters into bowls, using a slotted spoon, leaving the juice in the saucepan. Bring to the boil, then turn the heat down to low and simmer for a few minutes until the juice is syrupy.

3 Remove from the heat and stir to allow the mixture to cool slightly, then stir in the crème fraîche and mix with the nectarines. Sprinkle over the orange zest and serve.

Nutrition facts (per serving)
Calories 144   Carbohydrate 22g   Protein 1.2g   Fat 4g (of which saturates 4g)

Berry Meringues Serves 4

Preparation time: 5 minutes

These seem to be a hit with adults and children alike and offer you a simple and quick way to make strawberries a bit more exciting.

4 meringue nests
250g/9oz strawberries, hulled and chopped
4 scoops of Frozen Vanilla Yogurt (see page 200)

Put the meringue nests on serving plates and divide the chopped strawberries between them – don't worry if some are tumbling over the sides. Top with a scoop of Frozen Vanilla Yogurt and serve.

Nutrition facts (per serving)
Calories 160   Carbohydrate 30g   Protein 11.4g   Fat 0g (of which saturates 0g)

Greek-Style Potted Lemon Cheesecake Serves 4

Preparation time: 10 minutes

If you are following a strict training plan and trying to fuel accordingly, standard cheesecake would be difficult to validate. However, this makes a much lighter option, with the added benefits of being high in protein, essential fatty acids, vitamin E, calcium, phosphorus and magnesium.

4 tbsp Nut Butter, made with almonds
  (see page 131)
zest and juice of ½ lemon

4 tsp lemon curd
400g/14oz fat-free Greek yogurt

1 Put 1 tablespoon Nut Butter at the bottom of four individual dessert bowls, tall glasses or goblets.

2 In a large bowl, mix together the lemon juice, lemon curd and yogurt until well blended. Layer this yogurt mix over the top of each almond butter base and smooth the top. Sprinkle with the lemon zest, cover and chill in the fridge until ready to serve.

Nutrition facts (per serving)
Calories 179   Carbohydrate 8.2g   Protein 14g   Fat 11g (of which saturates 1.9g)

Rhubarb Granola Crumble Serves 4

Preparation time: 15 minutes **Cooking time:** 10 minutes

Fruit crumble is a favourite with many people. This recipe removes the stodgier, higher-fat traditional topping and replaces it with a slow-release carbohydrate option, which is useful when aiming to fuel up for an endurance or high-intensity session the following morning.

4–6 rhubarb stalks, cut into small chunks
1 tbsp caster/granulated sugar

1 tsp mixed/apple pie spice
60g/2¼oz/½ cup granola

1 **Preheat the oven to 150°C/300°F/Gas 2.**

2 **Put the rhubarb and sugar in a saucepan with about 3 tablespoons water and cook over a low heat for about 8 minutes, or until the rhubarb is soft. Spoon the fruit into four small ovenproof dishes. Sprinkle over the mixed/apple pie spice and top with the granola.**

3 **Bake for 10 minutes until you see the fruit bubbling out the sides. Serve straight away.**

Nutrition facts (per serving)
Calories 100   Carbohydrate 15g   Protein 3g   Fat 3.7g (of which saturates 0.8g)

HERO FOOD: OATS

We've all been told time and time again how porridge/oatmeal is the best start to the day. It is low in fat, high in soluble fibre and is also a great source of complex carbohydrate. This means that it releases energy slowly throughout the day, preventing blood-sugar fluctuations or energy crashes. That said, oats don't necessarily need to be eaten as porridge/oatmeal. You can eat them cold in the form of Bircher or standard muesli or why not try an Oaty Banana Pancake (see page 135). You could also try oatcakes or even make your own energy bars (see page 188) to have as a snack pre- or during training. Whichever way, they should definitely be on your list as a go-to food to fuel long endurance training sessions.

Coconut & Mango Rice Pudding

Serves 4

Preparation time: 10 minutes   **Cooking time:** 30 minutes

I often recommend rice pudding to my athletes as a recovery choice. The milk content ensures that it has the ideal mix of carbohydrate and protein to repair and recover tired muscles. This recipe is a far cry from the sloppy rice pudding served at school with a dollop of jam!

400ml/14fl oz/generous 1½ cups reduced-fat canned coconut milk
450ml/16fl oz/scant 2 cups skimmed milk
75g/3oz/⅓ cup short-grain pudding rice

55g/2oz/¼ cup caster/granulated sugar
grated zest of 2 limes
juice of 1 lime
1 mango, peeled, pitted and sliced

1 Pour the coconut milk and milk into a saucepan and bring to the boil over a high heat. Turn the heat down to low and add the rice, sugar and lime zest. Simmer gently for about 20 minutes until the rice is soft and has absorbed most of the milk.

2 Meanwhile, drizzle the lime juice over the mango slices and toss together to coat.

3 Spoon the rice pudding into serving bowls and serve hot with the mango slices.

Nutrition facts (per serving)
Calories 252   Carbohydrate 50g   Protein 5.2g   Fat 5.2g (of which saturates 4.8g)

Poached Pears with Cardamom Custard Serves 4

Preparation time: 5 minutes   **Cooking time:** 15 minutes

Custard is often overlooked as a dessert these days, but it is an excellent way to ensure you meet your dairy requirements. I have made the custard the main feature in this recipe for that reason and added the poached pears as an accompaniment.

4 ripe pears, peeled, cored and halved
2 tbsp custard powder
500ml/17fl oz/2 cups skimmed milk

1 tbsp caster/granulated sugar
4 cardamom pods

1 Preheat the oven to 150°C/300°F/Gas 2.

2 Put the pear halves in a baking pan with just enough water to cover the base of the pan. Bake for 20 minutes, or until the pears are tender.

3 Meanwhile, make the custard. Put the custard powder in a measuring jug and add 1 tablespoon of the milk to make a paste. Put the rest of the milk, the sugar and cardamom pods in a saucepan and bring to the boil over a high heat.

4 Pour the milk mixture onto the custard paste in the measuring jug, whisking continuously so they blend completely without forming any lumps. Pour the contents of the jug back into the saucepan, turn the heat down to low and cook for about 5 minutes, stirring continuously, until the custard is thick

5 Pour the custard over the pears and serve hot.

Nutrition facts (per serving)
Calories 215   Carbohydrate 50g   Protein 5g   Fat 0g (of which saturates 0g)

GLOSSARY

acetyl co-enzyme A (acetyl-CoA) is an important molecule in metabolism, used in many biochemical reactions.

adenosine triphosphate (ATP) is a molecule that transports chemical energy within cells for metabolism.

adipose tissue is the scientific term for fat stores.

aerobic metabolism involves the production of energy via biochemical pathways in the presence of oxygen.

alpha-linolenic acid (ALA) is an essential omega-3 fatty acid necessary for growth and development.

amino acids – protein plays a crucial role in almost all biological processes and amino acids are the building blocks of it. Branched-chain amino acids are essential nutrients that the body obtains from proteins found in food – especially meat, dairy products and legumes. They include leucine, isoleucine and valine. 'Branched-chain' refers to the chemical structure of these amino acids.

anaerobic metabolism involves the production of energy via biochemical pathways in the absence of oxygen.

antioxidants are enzymes or other organic substances, such as vitamin E or beta-carotene, capable of counteracting the damaging effects of oxidation in animal tissues.

autoimmune condition – your body's immune system protects you from disease and infection. But if you have an autoimmune disease, your immune system attacks healthy cells in your body by mistake. Autoimmune diseases can affect many parts of the body.

beta-alanine is a naturally occurring amino acid used in athletes to help reduce acid levels when exercising at high intensity.

bioelectrical impedance testing is a commonly used method for estimating body composition, and in particular body fat.

body composition is the term used to measure levels of fat mass and non-fat mass. It is often expressed as body fat percentage.

Borg Scale – the recognized scale for measuring the level of exertion.

BW stands for body weight. In sports nutrition, calculations are worked out per kg of body weight.

cardiovascular system is an organ system that circulates blood, transporting nutrients, oxygen, carbon dioxide, hormones and blood cells to and from cells in the body to nourish it and help to fight diseases, stabilize body temperature and pH, and to maintain homeostasis.

co-enzymes are organic molecules that are required by certain enzymes to carry out reactions.

co-factors are often classified as inorganic substances that are required for, or increase the rate of, reactions.

creatine phosphate (CP) is a molecule that provides a rapidly transferable reserve of high energy into muscles and the brain.

curcumin is the principle component of the spice turmeric and a powerful antioxidant.

delayed onset muscle soreness (DOMS) is the pain and stiffness felt in muscles several hours to days after unaccustomed or strenuous exercise.

DHA, or docosahexaenoic acid, is an omega-3 fatty acid that is a primary structural component of the human brain.

electrolytes refers to salts such as sodium, potassium, magnesium etc. that are needed by the working muscle during exercise. Sodium and potassium help to

draw water in and prevent dehydration, while magnesium is necessary for muscle contraction.

enzymes are biological macro molecules that are responsible for thousands of metabolic processes that sustain life.

EPA, or eicosapentaenoic acid, is an omega-3 fatty acid found in fish oils and shown to help reduce inflammation and reduce cholesterol levels.

ergogenic aids are any external substances, such as caffeine, that can be determined to enhance performance in high-intensity exercises.

fatty acids make up the acid part of a fat molecule and can be either saturated or unsaturated.

fasted state when you have not eaten for a period of more than 6 hours.

fast-twitch muscle fibres are good for rapid movements like jumping to catch a ball or sprinting for the bus. They contract quickly, but get tired fast, as they consume lots of energy.

fat adapted – a method of eating and training that helps to improve the efficiency of using fat as fuel for endurance events.

follicular phase refers to the time of your menstrual cycle leading up to ovulation.

free radicals are atoms or groups of atoms and can be formed when oxygen interacts with certain molecules. Once formed, these highly reactive radicals can start a chain reaction, like dominoes. Their chief danger comes from the damage they can do when they react with important cellular components such as DNA, or the cell membrane.

GI (glycaemic index) is a rating system for foods containing carbohydrates. It shows how quickly each food affects your blood sugar (glucose) level when that food is eaten on its own.

glycogen is the body's store of glucose in muscles and liver when glucose is not needed at that moment in time. Glycogen is readily converted to glucose and transported to the working muscles on demand by the body.

glycolysis is the breakdown of glucose by enzymes into pyruvic and lactic acids, releasing energy in the absence of oxygen.

gluconeogenesis is the breakdown of non carbohydrate substrates such as fatty acids (fats) and amino acids (protein) to produce glucose for energy when there is not sufficient carbohydrate available.

glucose is a simple sugar and the principle source of energy for all living organisms.

gluten – protein found in wheat responsible for giving wheat dough its elastic nature.

haemoglobin is the iron-containing oxygen-transport protein in the red blood cells. Haemoglobin in the blood carries oxygen from the respiratory organs (lungs or gills) to the rest of the body (i.e. the tissues).

isoflavanoids are a classification of anti-oxidants.

lactate – a waste product of anaerobic respiration that accumulates in muscles during exercise.

lactate threshold – the point at which the levels of lactate in the blood are too high to be cleared by the oxygen available during exercise.

luteal phase is the period of time in the menstrual cycle post ovulation.

macronutrients are energy-providing chemical substances consumed by organisms in large quantities. The three macronutrients in nutrition are carbohydrates, lipids and proteins.

metabolic rate refers to the rate of energy expenditure.

micronutrients are nutrients required by humans and other organisms throughout life in small quantities.

mitochondria are the 'powerhouse of the cell' because they generate most of the cell's supply of adenosine triphosphate (ATP).

mmol (millimole) a unit of measurement equivalent to 1/1000 of a mole where a mole is 1 molecule.

motor control is the process by which humans and animals use their neuromuscular system to activate and co-ordinate the muscles and limbs involved in the performance of a motor skill

muscle contraction refers to the shortening or tensing of muscle fibres.

muscle hypertrophy refers to increasing the size of muscle fibres within a muscle.

muscle mass is the term used when talking about the amount of muscle within a body.

muscle protein synthesis is the building of muscle.

myocytes are the structural cells of a muscle.

myofibrils are the contractile fibre within muscle.

neuro-muscular system is the collective term for the muscles of the body, together with the nerves supplying them.

osteoporosis is a disorder in which the bones become increasingly porous, brittle and subject to fracture, owing to loss of calcium and other mineral components.

oxidative stress is damage to cell membranes within the body caused by free radicals.

phytates are a component of some high-fibre foods, including many cereal grains, which may, in excessive amounts, cause constipation or interfere with the body's ability to absorb minerals.

plyometrics is a system of dynamic muscle exercise, designed to develop power for running, jumping and throwing sports. It is based on the principle that muscles contract faster and with greater force when worked from a pre-stretched position.

polyphenols are organic compounds responsible for the colour and flavour of some fruits and vegetables; they may have antioxidant properties.

protein pulsing is the term used in sports nutrition when describing consumption of 0.25g/kg BW protein at regular intervals through the day to maximize muscle protein synthesis.

pyruvate is the end product of glycolysis and may be metabolized to lactate or to acetyl CoA.

rate of perceived exertion (RPE) is a scale used to measure the intensity of exercise. The RPE scale runs from 0–10 where 0 is being still and 10 is maximal intensity.

resynthesize is when depleted stores such as glycogen are rebuilt post exercise.

turbo session is a high-intensity bike session done indoors. The bike is attached to a platform so that it stays stationary while the individual can complete a workout.

BIBLIOGRAPHY

http://www.anorexiabulimiacare.org.uk/

Aragon, Alan Albert and Schoenfeld, Brad Jon, 'Nutrient timing revisited: is there a post-exercise anabolic window?', *Journal of the International Society of Sports Nutrition*, 2013

Burke, Louise, *Clinical Sports Nutrition*, 4th edition, 2010, McGraw-Hill Medical Publishing

Burke, Louise, *Practical Sports Nutrition*, 2007, Human Kinetics Publishing

Burke, Louise, et al., 'Nutrition for athletes, a position paper by nutrition working group of the IOC, International Olympic Committee', 2012

Deldicque, Louise and Francaux, Marc, 'Recommendations for healthy nutrition in female endurance runners: an update', *Frontiers in Nutrition*, May 2015, Vol. 2, article 17

Drobinic, F., et al., 'Reduction of delayed onset muscle soreness by a novel curcumin delivery system (Meriva®): a randomised, placebo-controlled trial', *Journal of the International Society of Sports Nutrition*, June 18, 2014

Eddy, Kate, *Strength and Conditioning*, colleague's notes – unpublished, 2014

Fuhrman, Dr Joel, et al , 'Fuelling the vegetarian (vegan) athlete', *Current Sports Medicine: Reports*, 2010, Vol. 9, No. 4

Gleeson, et al, 'Effect of probiotic on URTI incidence in an athlete cohort', *International Journal of Sports Nutrutrition and Exercise Metabolism*, 2011, 21 (1): 55–64

Gluek, C. J., et al., 'Severe vitamin D deficiency, myopathy and rhabdomyolysis', *North American Journal of Medical Sciences*, August 2013, volume 5, issue 8

Hausswirth, Christophe, et al., 'Physiological and nutritional aspects of post-exercise recovery specific recommendations for female athletes', *Sports Medicine Journal*, 2011, 41 (10): 861–882

Helms, Eric R., et al., 'A systematic review of dietary protein during caloric restriction in resistance trained lean athletes: A case for higher intakes', *International Journal of Sport Nutrition and Exercise*, September 2013

Isacco, L., et al., 'Influence of hormonal status on substrate utilization at rest and during exercise in the female population', *Sports Medicine Journal*: April 2012, 1;42 (4): 327–42

Jeukendrup, Asker, 'A step towards personalized sports nutrition: carbohydrate intake during exercise', *Sports Medicine Journal*, 2014, 44 (Suppl 1): S25–S33

Joy, Elizabeth, Kussman, Andrea and Nattiv, Aurelia, '2016 update on eating disorcers in athletes: A comprehensive narrative review with a focus on clinical assessment and management', *British Medical Journal*, January 2016

Kerksick, Chad et al., 'International Society of Sports Nutrition position stand: Nutrient timing', *Journal of the International Society of Sports Nutrition*, October 3, 2008

Łagowska, K., et al., 'Effects of dietary intervention in young female athletes with menstrual disorders', *Journal of the International Society of Sports Nutrition*, 2014, 11:21

Lenn, J. et al., 'The effects of fish oil and isoflavones on delayed onset muscle soreness', *Medical Science, Sports and Exercise*, Octobober 2002; 34 (10): 1605–13

Oosthuyse, T., et al., 'The effect of the menstrual cycle on exercise metabolism: implications for exercise performance in eumenorrhoeic women', *Sports Medicine Journal*, March 2010, 1;40 (3): 207–27

Phillips, Stuart M., 'Dietary protein requirements and adaptive advantages in athletes', *British Journal of Nutrition*, 2012, 108, S158–S167

Phillips, Stuart M., 'Protein consumption and resistance exercise: maximizing anabolic potential', *Sports Science Exchange*, 2013, Vol. 26, No. 107, 1–5

Phillips, Stuart M., et al., 'The role of milk- and soy-based protein in support of muscle protein synthesis and muscle protein accretion in young and elderly persons', *Journal of the American College of Nutrition*, 2009, Vol. 28, No. 4, 343–354

Pyne, D.B. et al., 'Probiotic supplementation for athletes – clinical and physiological effects', *European Journal of Sport Science*, 15 (1): 63–72

Spriet, Lawrence L., 'New insights into the interaction of carbohydrate and fat metabolism during exercise', *Sports Medicine Journal*, 2014, 44 (Suppl 1): S87–S96

Stark, Matthew, et al., 'Protein timing and its effects on muscular hypertrophy and strength in individuals engaged in weight-training', *Journal of the International Society of Sports Nutrition*, 2012, 9:54

Trexler, Eric T., Smith-Ryan, Abbie E. and Norton, Layne E., 'Metabolic adaptation to weight loss: implications for the athlete', *Journal of the International Society of Sports Nutrition*, 2014

Wardle, Katie R.D., et al., 'The nutritional demands of ultra-endurance running', www.ultrarunningltd.co.uk/training-schedule/nutrition/nutritional-demands-of-ultra-running

Williams, N.I., et al., 'Evidence for a causal role of low energy availability in the induction of menstrual cycle disturbances during strenuous exercise training', *The Journal of Clinical Endocrinology & Metabolism*, 2001: 86:5184–93

Wilmore, J.H. and Costill, D.L., *Physiology of Sport and Exercise*, 3rd edition, 2005, Human Kinetics Publishing

INDEX

ACKNOWLEDGMENTS

Once again I need to say a huge thanks to Watkins Media and Nourish books for all their support and advice, but in particular to Jo Lal, who had the original concept of fast fuel and Rebecca Woods, who has patiently listened and provided me with direction.

No book can be written without creativity and inspiration. I feel fortunate to be surrounded by so many amazing triathletes – you've all helped in your own way to produce this book.

I also need to say a special thank you to my beautiful daughters Maya and Ella who have had to put up with a very distracted mother for several months and late evening meals while I just write one more paragraph! And of course I must not forget my side kick, running buddy and Spaniel, Bailey – we've run for miles over the last few months, coming up with new ideas to keep this book fresh and interesting!

Thank you also to my ever patient husband, Andrew – I hope one day all this writing will pay off and you can sail away and have your own adventure! And also to the rest of my immediate family for putting up with weeks of me being distracted and spending hours in front of my laptop when I should have been conversing and catching up with you!

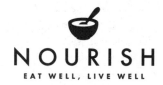

NOURISH
EAT WELL, LIVE WELL

Here at Nourish we're all about wellbeing through food and drink – irresistible dishes with a serious good-for-you factor. If you want to eat and drink delicious things that set you up for the day, suit any special diets, keep you healthy and make the most of the ingredients you have, we've got some great ideas to share with you. Come over to our blog for wholesome recipes and fresh inspiration – nourishbooks.com